TOXIC HOME/
CONSCIOUS HOME

This book is a "must-read" for everyone, whether you suffer from an 'unknown illness, or you just want to feel better and live a healthier life. From the water we drink to the energy that surrounds us, Dr. Rob Brown fills in special details about the numerous toxins in our environment — toxins we 'intuitively' sense. Written with elegant simplicity and humorous auto-biographical insight, Toxic Home is inspiring and motivating, giving us the tools we need to be a full participant in creating health. It's an invitation you dare not refuse."

Winter Robinson

Medical intuitive and author of Intuitions: *Seeing with the Heart and A Hidden Order: Uncover Your Life's Design*

"As an expert in the health effects of MRI for the past 30 years, I found Rob Brown's book very informative and useful. In it, he provides well researched and comprehensive coverage of many toxins found in the home and offers important tips for remediation, including the invisible and nearly ubiquitous EMF radiation. This book will be my go-to resource for eradicating these dangerous pollutants from my home in the future. "

Larry Burk, MD, CEHP

Author: *Let Magic Happen: Adventures in Healing with a Holistic Radiologist*

TOXIC HOME/
CONSCIOUS HOME

A Mindful Approach to Wellness at Home

ROB BROWN, MD

TOXIC HOME/CONSCIOUS HOME:
A Mindful Approach to Wellness at Home
Copyright © 2018 Rob Brown, MD.

Books may be ordered through booksellers or by contacting:

Healthy Berry, LLC
P. O. Box 299
Murrysville, PA 15668
724-552-7258
robbrownmd@gmail.com
http://robbrownmd.com

Because of the dynamic nature of the Internet, any web addresses or links contained in this book may have changed since publication and may no longer be valid. The views expressed in this work are solely those of the author and do not necessarily reflect the views of the publisher, and the publisher hereby disclaims any responsibility for them.

The author of this book does not dispense medical advice or prescribe the use of any technique as a form of treatment for physical, emotional, or medical problems without the advice of a physician, either directly or indirectly. The intent of the author is only to offer information of a general nature to help you in your quest for emotional and spiritual well- being. In the event you use any of the information in this book for yourself, which is your constitutional right, the author and the publisher assume no responsibility for your actions.

ISBN: 978-0-9997131-1-2 (sc)
ISBN: 978-0-9997131-0-5 (e)

Healthy Berry, LLC First Edition: January 31, 2018

Contents

Acknowledgments

Toxic Home/Conscious Home was an encompassing project that took several years to complete and required the participation and encouragement of many players. I am grateful to those who helped to make this book a reality.

I give thanks to my family, in particular my mother, now passed, who inspired me with her unwavering pursuit of good health. My sisters, Marj and Jackie, whose love and trust over the years provided me with the confidence to step out of the confinement of conventional medicine. I thank my children, Arthur and Ursula, for their love and for keeping me in touch with the concerns of the up-and-coming generation.

Thanks to Rita Pollock, James Lyons, and Gracie Lyons for taking their time to read through my rough, rough draft. I am appreciative of their encouragement and guidance toward improvements in style and content.

I am grateful to my editors Anne Dillon, Jason Buccholz, and my life-long friend, David Itkin, whose efforts helped make this material read smoothly and consistently.

Kathy Soroka, I have treasured your continuous support throughout this project and your inspiration for a suitable book title.

Thank you, Rebekkah Narli, for reading the manuscript and for using your creativity and passion to select a beautiful image for each chapter. Your amazing artistic talent brought this project to a whole new level.

Many thanks are given to Yvonne Kohano whose publishing experience, guidance and attention to detail has helped to transform my manuscript into a book.

Finally, I am obliged to Carol Duffy, Marilyn Masciantonio Morrison, and the staff at Norwin Hills - Excela Square Medical Center for their support and encouragement. You all made this journey so much fun and truly rewarding.

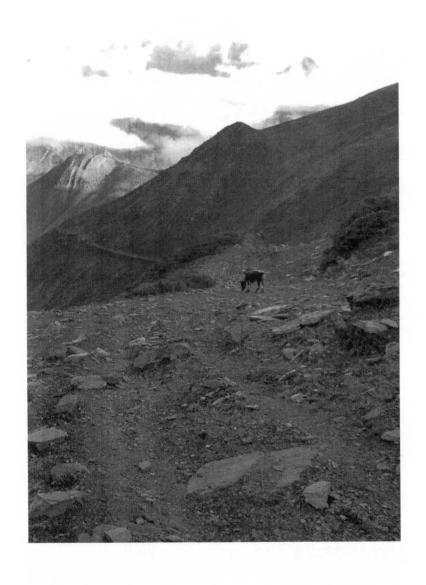

Introduction

Despite living in comfortable residences with climate control, refrigeration, plush beds, various modes of entertainment, and an assortment of personal devices, an increasing number of people in the US are maximally stressed and suffer from chronic illness. The incidence of health conditions such as asthma, heart disease, obesity, and neurodegenerative diseases is increasing at an alarming rate.[1,2]

Conscious choices are decisions you make based on understanding and knowledge. Creating a conscious home refers to making educated choices that will preserve and increase the well-being of the home's occupants. To optimize your health, it's critical to evaluate your personal environment. Aside from cleanliness, the goal in creating a healthy home is to maintain an environment that represents an extension of your natural state of being.

As you work toward this goal, it is necessary to understand your physical and biochemical relationship to your surroundings. The human body is an organism composed of trillions of tiny subunits called cells, each of which work together to make your body function as a whole. Every day, billions of these cells are reproducing, while others are dying. The body is designed to repair itself constantly. At nighttime, in particular, the body's reparative mechanism goes into full swing, allowing one to wake up refreshed and healed in the morning. It is important to have a calm, relaxing place to rest at the end of each day so the body can heal itself. Without this refuge, your body can become overwhelmed with repair needs. The result of this is distress, and then disease.

From health to medicine

My initial exposure to the health field began as a child. The late sixties and seventies were a time when all kinds of new products and technologies were hitting the market. Processed foods became prevalent and there was an explosion of plastic and synthetic products. Our household didn't partake in many of the new trends. Instead of eating processed, prepackaged snacks at lunch, we were given pieces of fruit and cut-up vegetables. Once our milkman made his final run and stopped delivering milk to our back door, our mother began to buy milk from the market. But instead of drinking processed milk products, we were fed "raw" milk, purchased at a neighborhood "health food store."

My mother's passion for maintaining good health led her to become a silent pioneer in the field of wellness. Her emphasis was on what was then called "health food," a label used before the now-ubiquitous term "organic." The health world was in its infancy at the time. The biochemical effects of nutrients were incompletely understood. The microbiome had yet to be discovered and the potential dangers of the many industrial chemicals and plastics consumers were bringing into their homes were largely unknown.

Growing up in this health-conscious environment naturally led me to a career in the health care profession. Following college, I spent four years at medical school transforming into an American medical doctor. Our class initially studied the anatomy and physiology of the human body to prepare us to learn the mechanisms of disease, as they were understood at that time. We learned how to recognize and treat disease, but there was little emphasis on preventative health aside from screening exams for various diseases and vaccinations. There was no education on diet, health, or wellness in medical school.

For post-graduate training, I chose radiology, a field which allowed me to marry my interest in the visual arts with my medical background. A radiologist may look at a hundred or more examinations each workday and is privileged to see the anatomical and sometimes physiological effects of disease processes on every organ system, with perhaps the exception of skin. After seeing tens of thousands of examinations, the radiologist begins to develop judgment which then allows him or her to differentiate between what is normal, or at least common and not of any clinical concern, from conditions that need treatment or follow-up.

Moshi and magnets

After residency training and board certification, I took time to work and travel before starting a fellowship program. During that year, I worked part-time for a radiology group and during my time off, I travelled. The biggest undertaking of the year was an extended trip to East Africa during which I volunteered at a medical clinic in Moshi, Tanzania, teaching radiology to African physicians. Afterwards, I arranged to climb Mt. Kilimanjaro. The preparation for this trek became a pivotal experience that forever changed my perspective on medicine and the health care field.

Mt. Kilimanjaro is a tall mountain, towering 19,762 feet above the flat African savannah. It isn't technically a climb, but rather a really long walk. I spent many months training at a gym on a treadmill, which had been placed in a hypoxic (low oxygen) chamber, something that was trendy at the time. I slowly built up my endurance and decided to do a practice hike before the Africa adventure. My cousin Roberta and I chose to celebrate my thirtieth birthday together and do a "pre-climb" on Mt. Rainier in Washington state, three months before my scheduled African adventure. The weather was perfect and the hike was glorious. But halfway down the trail, I twisted my knee and it rapidly swelled. I limped the rest of the way with my cousin's assistance.

That night, as we soaked in an outdoor hot tub, to say that I was discouraged would be an understatement. My cousin and her friend, who had joined us, suggested that I try alternative treatments, such as arnica or acupuncture, for my knee. Roberta had spent many years in London and had become familiar with a different style of health care. I can look back at this time and ashamedly admit that I didn't see any value in her suggestions. I believed at that time that if I didn't have the answer, I at least knew where to look for it. After all, I had just completed medical school, a residency program, and passed my boards in the US medical system, the best medical system in the world! I spouted off that I was pretty sure I had torn my meniscus and that I was going to need to see an orthopedic surgeon when I got home. Roberta's friend didn't appreciate my arrogance and we ended up getting into a heated discussion about the US health system. The argument was so charged that my cousin feared we would not be speaking to each other in the morning. This discourse foreshadowed a manifestation soon to come.

Upon getting back home, I quickly went to an orthopedic surgeon who prescribed an anti-inflammatory. All I could think about was my trip to Africa and getting my knee in shape for the Kilimanjaro hike. The pills took away the pain and swelling, but when I tried to stop the pills after a six-week course, the pain quickly returned. Driving was particularly unnerving, for every time I pressed down on the clutch, I felt my knee twinge. The clock was ticking. I was supposed to fly to Africa in six weeks.

It was then that one of my coworkers, after watching me struggle to get up and down from my desk chair, cautiously asked me if I was willing to try an alternative treatment. It's important to understand that at that time in the medical field, anything nonconventional was pretty much considered quackery, regardless of whether or not it worked. I did not yet understand that the US medical system is a huge industry that exists not only to heal people, but also to make money and to destroy the competition, like any successful business. Anything not promoted by the industry was viciously discredited. Anyway, my colleague, also wearing an MD on his white jacket, risked his reputation and cautiously asked me if I was open-minded and willing to try something "kind of out there" for my knee pain. Although my curiosity was piqued, I began looking into canceling my trek.

After agreeing to the mysterious treatment, my colleague brought to work two small round metal discs, the size of half dollars, and taped one on either side of my afflicted knee. He told me that they were specially designed magnets and to leave them taped to my knee for a few days. During the day, my knee didn't feel any differently, but while driving home, I noticed that I didn't feel that twinge in my knee while I pressed down the clutch pedal.

The pain subsided rapidly and within a few days, as long as I wore the magnets, I had no pain at all. I wore those magnets daily from them on, and even climbed Kilimanjaro with them taped to my knee. I experienced no twinges or pain of any kind. And, let me add, this was not an easy trip. On the last day of the Kilimanjaro trek we hiked twenty-five miles, descending from 12,700 feet to the entrance gate at the base at 6,100 feet. I think back to that time now and I am so grateful to this doctor, and now friend, for piercing my bubble and introducing me to an alternative world of medicine.

After my initial healing with magnets, I shared my amazement with some of my old classmates and fellow residents, but most of them listened skeptically and considered my cure to have been a placebo effect. It was then that I understood that what we had all been told to accept and to reject in allopathic medical training was not 100% correct. I knew that if I hadn't used the magnets, I would have missed my trip and instead ended up in surgery for a meniscal tear. The surgery would have predisposed me to chronic knee problems later in life. In this case, an alternative treatment was clearly more effective than a conventional treatment. Roberta and her friend had been right that night on Mt. Rainier. I must admit it took me years to experiment with other treatment options, including acupuncture and chiropractic manipulation. And, over the years, I have experienced superb healing with these techniques too.

From medicine back to health

After my year of exploration, I sub-specialized within radiology and studied musculoskeletal radiology in a fellowship program. This seemed like a relevant field of study for me as I had always been fascinated by sports-related injuries. I studied with leaders in the field and subsequently worked in many different medical practice settings, including at academic institutions, in private practice groups, and on the road as a traveling physician. I learned to appreciate the work of academicians who advance the field and gained respect for their contemporaries in private practice. Each practice opportunity provided me with a view into the surrounding community's health status. In this regard, the most interesting period of my career was during my tenure as a traveling physician.

I had the opportunity to work in many different settings and spend time in cities and small towns all over the US. Different types of diseases were more prevalent in different areas. Some communities had an exorbitant number of miscarriages while other areas had a large number of cases of neurodegenerative disease, such as multiple sclerosis. Chronic lung diseases were more prevalent in some regions, while others seemed to have a larger- than-expected number of bizarre, uncommon cancers. I even noticed that some areas had more disorders such as kidney stones and deposits of calcification in tendons, ligaments, and joints, which seemed to vary not only by location, but also by season. Obesity prevalence also varied, and some towns had larger populations of people who appeared to be very healthy.

I came to understand firsthand that diseases are not randomly distributed. In other words, the area where you live affects your chance of getting sick with a given disease. Our genes influence our expression of disease, but the environment, whether because of temperature, humidity, latitude, or a human-induced environmental toxin or toxicant, has a real influence on people. Sometimes we discover a source of toxicity in a community, but this is rare. The lead poisoning incident in Flint, MI that arose in 2016 is one such example. This was a tragic misfortune for the members of the Flint community, but lead poisoning has occurred before and will occur again. Furthermore, lead is only one of numerous potential contaminants that can affect human health. Another highly publicized incident was that uncovered by Erin Brockovich in which a power company had contaminated water supplies with hexavalent chromium, a toxic heavy metal that caused terrible misfortune to the surrounding communities. It's hard to believe, but hexavalent chromium is still found at unsafe levels in many municipal water systems in this country.

The increasing prevalence of environmental toxins has contributed to health problems for almost all of us. Why are we all living with so many toxins? One answer might be that we live in a country where the law states that we are presumed innocent until proven guilty. This concept applies to people as well as to products and the companies that produce them. Aside from the initial testing a product goes through in a lab, in our country, the burden of proving that a product is harmful is on the populace, and not on the company. A toxic, harmful product may be on the market for many years before enough data has been collected and the evidence becomes indisputable that the product is indeed causing disease. Add to this the misinformation created by marketing firms designed to blur facts and it has become very difficult to prove that any products in the marketplace are harmful at all.

The tendency of industry to promote new technology at the expense of human health is nothing new. Consider that the danger of radiation was known in 1927, yet it wasn't until 1970 that radiation boxes, which allowed children in shoe stores to see their toes wiggle inside their shoes and were marketed as providing the "best possible fit," were finally banned in thirty-three states. As a radiologist I find this particularly disturbing, knowing the requirements for lead shielding and quality control to operate an X-ray machine and fluoroscope in the medical imaging field today.

We may not realize toxic effects when a product initially comes to market, but if toxicity becomes evident over time, there will be resistance to removing the product from the marketplace, especially if the product is popular. It would be best if governments and businesses always did the right thing and removed products with harmful toxins, regardless of the hassle and cost, but this isn't the case. Media, research, and government policy are influenced by the broad reach of multinational corporations through ownership and lobbying power and as a result, most people in this country and in the world at large have very little knowledge of what is hazardous to their health. Add the influx of international products with their own largely unknown potential toxins, and we have ended up with significant toxin burdens in our homes. Contaminants in our environment are accumulating at an alarming rate, and the hazards we face daily continue to become more confusing and diverse.

What is the difference between a toxin and toxicant?

Before the explosion of industrially produced chemicals in our society, toxins were initially described as agents that cause harm to the body in small amounts. Now, the term toxin is usually reserved for naturally occurring elements such as lead, mercury, and arsenic as well as poisons produced by plants and animals. The term toxicant is used when referring to potentially harmful human-engineered chemical agents, which are present in everything from your lunch meat to plastic wrap and suntan lotion. But knowledge and lifestyle changes can help reduce household exposure to both toxins and toxicants.

Toxins and toxicants can affect our health. Although we may not be able to detect them with our five senses, it is important to understand that our relationship to the environment is not limited to our senses. An object or experience detectable by the senses may seem more real. But, forces that we are unable to sensibly perceive are constantly interacting with our bodies, though we might be oblivious to them.

Have you ever walked into a room and suddenly, your eyes water? You may sneeze as your body's immune system kicks into hyperdrive because somewhere in the local environment there is something your body is allergic to. In many instances, your body senses an allergen that cannot be seen, smelled, or felt. Have you ever felt antsy or irritable when in a specific room for no apparent reason? What are you sensing in this situation? A feeling of irritability may be some form of nervous system reaction to an environmental stimulus. Depending on our presence and "in-tune-ness" we can become aware of many things. If you become more conscious, the evidence is everywhere.

What you will learn by reading Toxic Home/Conscious Home

Each chapter in this book explores a distinct realm within the home. After providing a bit of background information, I emphasize what you can do to minimize your toxin/toxicant exposure and optimize your health. The first three chapters deal with the essentials of life, food, air, and water. These are the most important areas to start with for they are crucial for sustainable life. From there, the book will take a look at those things in your home that make living easier and more pleasant. Processed foods, packaging materials, personal care products, artificial sources of light, and sound are potential sources of convenience and enjoyment, but can also infuse toxic elements into the home and as such bear discussion. The final section is dedicated to unseen, immeasurable undercurrents within your home. The ancient Chinese discipline *feng shui* and the elusive effects of meditation will help you to create a beautiful home that reflects who you are within, and also give you an idea of what you can create in your world outside the home.

This book is geared towards those who like to experiment and to try out new ideas, and especially for those who are looking for ways to improve their health and the health of their families. Reducing the toxin and toxicant load from the home does not necessarily mean one must give up modern conveniences or entertainment. But with some modification to lifestyle, it will be easier to rest peacefully at night and stay well. As you slowly work your way through this book, steadily making a lifestyle change here and there, you will find one day that you are living in a happier, healthier place.

PART I
ESSENTIALS

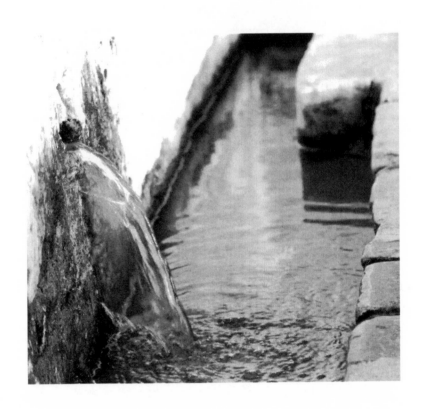

Chapter 1

WATER

I began an in-depth study of water several years ago when the hydraulic fracturing ("fracking") boom hit the country. I was lucky (or unlucky, depending on whose side you're on) to be living above a vast reservoir of underground natural gas, a highly sought-after area for fracking. Having enjoyed clean well water for many years, I was suddenly faced with the possibility of having my ground water contaminated.

At the time, the industry and governmental regulatory agencies denied that such a thing could possibly happen, but I proceeded to study water systems and all of the water filters on the market to see which of them would remove the most contaminants. I didn't have access to a list of potential toxins associated with fracking—the industry is not required to disclose that information to the public—but I had heard rumors that salts and volatile organic compounds (VOCs), such as benzene and xylene, were frequently used in fracking fluid. So I searched for filters that would remove these compounds and others. I learned that although there is a great difference among the various filtration systems in the marketplace, no filters are capable of removing all contaminants.

What is water?

Water is an amazing liquid material composed of H_2O (two hydrogen atoms and one oxygen atom) molecules. These molecules can actually function as tiny dipole magnets. One side of the molecule, the oxygen atom, has a negative charge, while the hydrogen side of the molecule has a positive charge. Water molecules align themselves with each other and with other charged particles. By surrounding other charged particles, water molecules can incorporate and dissolve them into their magnetic lattice. Water is known as a universal solvent because it can dissolve more substances within it than any other liquid. Pure water has a neutral pH, meaning it is not acidic or alkaline. On the pH scale, which ranges from 1 to 14, pure water is 7.0.

Water also demonstrates cohesion, meaning that water molecules stick to one another. In addition, water has adhesive properties, in that water molecules are attracted to surfaces other than water. The combination of these two characteristics gives water a property called surface tension. This quality allows water to travel and move through tubes, such as blood vessels, as well as a plant's root system.

Pure water is odorless, tasteless, and a clear, transparent liquid. Importantly, water can absorb and transmit energy. We all see this in action when we go to the beach and see the power of waves moving through water.

Pure water

Pure water (containing only H_2O molecules) does not naturally occur and can only be created by the processes of deionization and distillation. Distillation is the simpler concept to understand. In order to distill water, an impure source of water is boiled at 100°C (212°F), creating water steam. This water vapor is then condensed, cooled, and re-collected. All of the dissolved materials, such as salts, minerals, and other contaminants, which boil at a higher temperature, are left in the original container. However, dissolved substances that become gaseous and evaporate at a lower or similar temperature may sneak into the water vapor and contaminate the distillate.

The creation of deionized water involves a multistep process that includes reverse osmosis technology (described later in this chapter), and forcing water through a special deionization medium, which removes any remaining ions (charged atoms and molecules). The water produced by deionization is typically purer than distilled water.

As pure water is exposed to the environment, it will immediately begin the process of incorporating and dissolving materials from the surrounding environment. Materials that dissolve within the liquid will then move through water via a process called diffusion. Imagine placing a drop of dye in one end of a tank of water. At first, the coloring is most intense at the area of application, but over time, the entire tank of water will become a homogeneous shade of pale color. Diffusion occurs with all types of gases and particulates in the overlying air as well as those compounds within the water's container.

Pure water can hydrate the body, but is not a source of nourishment and can be dangerous to living cells.[1] Through a chemical process called osmosis, pure water outside a cell will move through the membrane of a living cell, attempting to equalize the concentration of the salts within the cell with the pure water outside. This is an impossible task. Eventually, the cell will explode, a phenomenon referred to as lysis.

Natural states of water

On our planet, naturally occurring water is grouped into two categories: saline water and freshwater. The difference between these is determined by the amount of dissolved salts within the water, measured in parts per million (ppm). Water is classified as freshwater if the total measured amount of dissolved salts is less than 1000 ppm. This means that in freshwater, less than 0.1% of the water's weight comes from dissolved salts. Water is saline if it has more than 1000 ppm of dissolved salts.

When salt is added to water, the salt's atoms and molecules split apart. The resulting atoms and molecules carry positive or negative charges and are referred to as ions. The most common ions found in water from the dissolution of salts include sodium, potassium, magnesium, calcium, chloride, and sulfate. Varying concentrations of all these salts are necessary for life.

Most (>96%) of the world's water is saline. Saline water fills the world's oceans, bays, and estuaries. Saline can also be found naturally within groundwater, and is very common in the western US. But humans and most animals require freshwater for drinking. Why is this? Although our bodies are composed of mostly salt water, the concentration of salts in the blood is tightly regulated by our kidneys and circulating hormones. Our bodies create this special internal environment by absorbing salts from food and mixing them with the freshwater that we drink. In this way, our blood can act as a reservoir of the proper fluid for our cells, creating microenvironments of varying salt concentrations. This maintains our cells' abilities to perform their specific tasks. Many important chemical reactions within the body require specific salt concentrations. For example, a nerve cell is able to transmit an impulse by the movement of salts in and out of the length of the cell.

Excess salts and/or excess water are excreted out of your body through urine created by your kidneys. If you drink a large volume of saline water, your body may become too "salty" and may not be able to maintain its internal homeostasis. Death can occur if salt levels in the blood go too high.

Freshwater exists on Earth in several different naturally occurring forms, including lakes and ponds, flowing rivers and streams, and as ground water. Water vapor and rain complete the fresh water cycle. Rain water falls to the ground and percolates through the soil and rocks until it reaches the water table, the depth at which the rock material is saturated with water. Some ground water sources, called aquifers, can be readily retrieved by digging wells or accessing springs.

Ground water slowly moves downhill and may then seep into rivers, streams, lakes, and the ocean. Water evaporates from these bodies of water, coalesces into droplets, and becomes rain again. Freshwater also evaporates from animals during perspiration and from plants during transpiration. Large forests, such as the Amazon rainforest, actually create their own weather patterns of rainfall due to the extensive water vapor in the air that accumulates from transpiration.

Freshwater is often stored in reservoirs for a population's water consumption. A reservoir can be a natural lake or a man-made body of water. Dams are often constructed in river valleys to block the flow of water, creating reservoirs. Earth can also be excavated and lined by walls and levees to contain the water within.

Given these various methods for accessing freshwater, it is important to understand what we want and what we don't want in our water to optimize our health and prevent disease. For optimal health, our drinking and bathing water should be either neutral or slightly basic in pH and should have some salts dissolved within it, as well as trace amounts of the minerals our bodies need, such as calcium and magnesium.[2]

Proper pH is important and should be considered a top priority when evaluating drinking water. Acidic water, which is water with a pH lower than 7, will dissolve higher concentrations of minerals, heavy metals, and other contaminants than will water with a slightly higher pH.[3,4] The increased dissolution of contaminants can lead to toxicity. Although contamination may originate from the water's source, heavy metals, particularly lead, may also leach from pipes carrying water to its destination.[5] Alkaline water, which is water with a pH higher than 7, can be bitter in taste and can also dissolve metals and other compounds. Alkaline water can cause the crusting of deposits in appliances and can cause chlorine to lose its effectiveness, thereby requiring more for proper disinfection.[6]

Just as we can manipulate salt concentrations, different sections of our bodies, particularly our gastrointestinal tracts, are able to raise or lower local pH to optimize the function of specific proteins called enzymes. Many disease processes, especially those caused by inflammation, are exacerbated by lower pH, and can sometimes be ameliorated by drinking water that is slightly alkaline.[7]

Trace minerals are important for many of our physiological processes, such as the construction of proteins. For example, iron, an integral part of the blood cells' main functional protein, hemoglobin, is necessary for the cells' ability to carry oxygen and carbon dioxide. It has been reported that most Americans suffer from mineral deficiencies. Minerals and trace elements are only absorbed if they are in an ionic form, as they are when dissolved in water.

Water contaminants

So, what is it that we don't want in our drinking water? The list is long, but can be grouped into categories: salts, agricultural products, medications, radionuclides, petroleum products and volatile organic compounds (VOCs), disinfectants, microscopic pathogens (organisms that cause disease), excessive heavy metals, and sediment. Depending on your water source, any or all of these pollutants may be present. As cities have grown, water quality from local resources such as reservoirs and aquifers has deteriorated. Ground water will often contain more dissolved chemicals than surface water. It has been the government's role to protect rivers, streams, lakes, and aquifers, but the limits imposed on specific pollutants have been skewed in favor of industry.

Disinfectants are commonly added to water systems intentionally, but they may also accumulate in water supplies unintentionally. Chlorine is an inexpensive compound commonly added to drinking water systems to kill bacteria and other potential disease-causing microorganisms. Adding chlorine causes the removal of some trace elements, such as manganese and iron, from the water. Depending on its original composition, this may not be desirable in some water supplies.[8,9] Chlorine can be delivered to a water supply by adding disinfectants, chloramines, and chlorine dioxide to the water. These chemical disinfectants can break down into byproducts including trihalomethanes and haloacetic acid, which are known to cause health risks, including cancer.[10,11] In 1998, the EPA set limits for the concentration of trihalomethane in drinking water due to its association with bladder cancer.[12] The World Health Organization has also set worldwide intake limits for most disinfectants and their byproducts.[13] However, many are concerned that the acceptable limits set by the EPA and WHO are too high.[14,15] It's a delicate balance, weighing the public health risk of widespread water-borne diseases against the increased risk of some individuals developing cancer from chemical disinfectants.

Your water source may also contain heavy metals such as lead, barium iron, mercury, manganese, magnesium, calcium, copper, selenium, zinc, arsenic, cadmium, or strontium, among others. Metals can enter the water system from several sources, including industrial sources and urban runoff. Emissions from coal-burning power plants, waste incineration, and industrial waste disposal may bring heavy metals into the waterways and water table. Although some metals, such as calcium, copper, zinc, and chromium, are required by the body in small quantities, large doses can be toxic. Lead, mercury, arsenic, and cadmium are a few heavy metals known to cause serious damage to the human body even in small quantities.[16]

Fluoride is a controversial additive in many public water systems around the country. It is introduced by adding the chemicals hydrofluorosilicic acid, sodium fluoride, or fluorosilicate to drinking supplies. Low levels of fluoride have been shown to aid in warding off dental cavities, particularly in children, but some have questioned the possible toxicities associated with this practice. Much like calcium, fluoride incorporates into skeletal bones and makes them harder, but fluoride, when ingested in high concentrations, causes dense bones that are weak and brittle, a disease known as fluorosis.

Fluorosis doesn't occur from the low levels of fluoride commonly placed into municipal water supplies. But communities in some countries have experienced fluorosis as a result of markedly elevated concentrations of fluoride in their drinking water after constructing wells that have tapped into water sources with too much dissolved fluoride from surrounding granite rocks.[17] There have been epidemiological studies to assess the potential dangers of lower concentrations of fluoride, but to date, no definite correlation has been determined between the ingestion of fluoride and the occurrence of cancer or other disease in humans.[18,19] Many cities across the US are saving money by no longer adding fluoride to their water systems.

Increased sediment, measured as total dissolved solids (TSS), will cause cloudiness, or turbidity, of the water. These particulates accumulate from the passage of water through silt, clay, and other sediments. Decomposing plants and animals as well as insoluble oxidized metals such as iron and manganese may contribute to water's turbidity.

There is a strong association between increased sediment and contaminated water. Sediment particles provide an attachment place for other pollutants, including heavy metals and bacteria. Bacteria attached to particulates in the water can be sheltered and protected from disinfectants, reducing their effectiveness.

Where does your water come from?

In the US, we are very fortunate to have a system of public works and private well water that provides most of the population with treated freshwater. Despite these two inexpensive, widely available drinking water sources, many people spend money on bottled water, thinking that the water they are purchasing is purer and healthier than the water coming out of their municipal water source or well.

Tap water

Do you drink your water straight from the tap? Most tap water comes directly from freshwater sources such as lakes, rivers, reservoirs, and aquifers. The water is first collected in a treatment plant to undergo sterilization and disinfection by chlorine. So the water you receive in your home should be free of bacteria and other organisms, but it can contain other contaminants.

The government has set up parameters for water safety, executed by the EPA and other federal agencies, to limit the concentration of some of these contaminants in the drinking water supply. Municipalities provide their citizenry with annual water test results that provide a basic analysis of their public water sources (Figure 1), but the tests are in no way inclusive of all the potential contaminants. If you look at the water test performed by my municipality, for example, you'll notice that of all the possible organic compounds known to infiltrate ground water from industrial processes, it only tests for two: trihalomethanes and haloacetic acids, the two chlorination byproducts regulated by the WHO and EPA! Volatile organic compounds (VOCs), both natural and industrial, can easily dissolve in water. Although there are hundreds, if not thousands of VOCs, only a small fraction of them are monitored and regulated by the EPA.

Figure 1. Water testing parameters

Typical Municipal Authority Test	Regulated VOCs not included in testing
INORGANIC CHEMICALS	**Benzene**
Copper	**1,4 Dichlorobenzene**
Lead	**Carbon Tetrachloride**
Nitrate	**Chlorobenzene**
Barium	**1,2-Dichlorobenzene**
Fluoride	**1,2-Dicholoroethane**
Mercury	**1,1-Dichloroethene**
Asbestos	**cis-1,2-Dichloroethene**
Total Chlorine Residual	**Trans-1,2 Dichloroethene**
Entry Point	**1,2-Dichloropropane**
ORGANIC CHEMICALS	**Ethylbenzene**
Total Trihalomethanes	**Methylene chloride**
Halo Acetic Acids	**Styrene**
TREATMENT TECHNIQUE	**Tetrachloroethene**
Turbidity	**Toluene**
Bacteria	**1,2,4-Trichlorobenzene**
Total Organic Carbon	**1,1,2-Trichloroethane**
RADIOACTIVE	**1,1,1-Trichloroethane**
Gross Alpha particles	**Trichlroethene**
Radium 226	**Vinyl Chloride**
Radium 228	**Xylene**
Total Uranium	
UNREGULATED	
Chromium	
Strontium	
Chlorate	

If you receive municipally treated water, you should check annually to find out if the water you are drinking and bathing in is contaminated with VOCs such as benzene or toluene. If you have a well, it is important to also test for methane. Independent water testing companies can provide a more complete evaluation of the water that comes from your faucet.

It is important to study these water test results. Consider that the maximum acceptable limits for contaminants are sometimes made with underlying political pressure by industry, and not necessarily for optimal public health. Given the extensive industry in many regions of the country, the maximum contaminant levels may represent a compromise of industry needs and the limited capability of water treatment plants to filter industrial chemicals from the water supply.

Regardless of your location, it is potentially dangerous to drink your tap water without any further filtering. If you choose to drink unfiltered tap water, especially if you haven't run the faucet in a few hours, run cold water through your pipes for twenty or thirty seconds before collecting water to drink. This will help allow any potential lead or other toxins that may have leached into your water over time from household pipes and tubing to be eliminated.[20] It is also best to draw cold water instead of hot water for drinking, as hot water can contain more heavy metals and other dissolved solutes within it than cold water.[21]

Well water

Whereas the recipient of municipal water is dependent on the utility company and government regulation for the quality of their water, the owner of a private well has the sole responsibility of ensuring the cleanliness of the water source. Typically, a well owner should assess water quality every year. Potential contaminants for a private well are the same as those for ground water in general and include hydrogen sulfide (sulfur), salt, and organic compounds, including methane gas, petroleum products, pesticides, fertilizers, biological wastes, septic system contaminants, and bacteria.

One of the benefits of well water is that it's free, aside from the energy required to run the pump and the materials needed for disinfection. But water analysis can be pricey, depending on which contaminants are surveyed. If your well water is contaminated, remediation may or may not be possible. For example, ground water contaminated by saline can be very difficult to remedy. Perhaps the greatest potential hazard for well owners is the presence of methane gas. If your well water contains dissolved methane gas, you need to install a special venting system for the water to prevent a possible explosion.

There are a few things you can do to help protect your well water. First of all, make sure that your septic system is distant enough from the well, and if you have livestock make sure their wastes are deposited far from the well head. Although many well owners install chlorination systems, it is best to limit the exposure of your water to this source of potential pathogens. While maintaining your property, try not to use any pesticides, fertilizers, or herbicides in the vicinity of your well head. Conventional pesticide and fertilizer residues can leach into the water table and persist for decades!

Bottled water

With few exceptions, purchasing bottled water is an unnecessary expense and a blight on the environment. The first time I saw a plastic water bottle for sale, I thought, "How ridiculous! Why would someone purchase water in a bottle?" How shortsighted I was. Bottled water is now a huge industry (Table 1).

Table 1. Most common companies selling spring water

Perrier (Vergèze, France)
Zephyrhills (Florida)
Nestlé (Erin, Ontario)
Fiji (Fiji)
Arrowhead (Nestlé company) (California)
Calistoga (Napa Valley, California)
Evian (Évian-les-Bains, France)
Crystal Geyser (California)
Glacier Mountain (Ohio)
Everest (Texas)
Poland Springs (Nestlé company) (One-third from Maine)

There are several different categories of bottled water in the market. These include distilled water, mineral water, purified water, sparkling water, and spring water. Bottled water is considered to be a food product and is therefore regulated by the FDA. According to regulations, bottled water must be 100% free of coliform bacteria and must be virtually lead- free. Interestingly, most municipal water sources will allow their water to contain up to three times more lead than is allowed in bottled water. Although this sounds like the bottled water industry is tightly regulated, it isn't. Believe it or not, the US municipal water regulations in general are much more stringent than the regulations for the bottled water industry. Aside from bacterial and lead content, the regulatory requirements for bottled water are sparse.

Two water sources provide bottling companies with their product. These are fresh springs and municipal or treated water systems. According to the EPA, water may be classified as spring water if it comes from a groundwater source that flows naturally to the earth's surface or from a well. Companies that bottle spring water are not required to disclose exactly where their water sources are located.

Naturally, the content and characteristics of spring waters vary depending on their sources. If the total number of dissolved solids in the water is greater than 250 ppm, the water is considered to be mineral water. Calistoga is a popular brand of mineral water. If water contains carbon dioxide (CO_2), it is labeled sparkling water. If CO_2 is lost from the water during processing, it may be added back at the same concentration it had when it emerged from its source and still be marketed as sparkling water. Perrier is a common brand of sparkling water.

Much of the bottled water sold in the US is taken directly from municipal water systems and purified prior to bottling. The two most popular brands of bottled water in this category are produced by the two rival cola companies, Coca-Cola and Pepsico. These bottles of repackaged water may not contain more than 10 ppm of dissolved solids and must be treated to remove chemicals and pathogens through distillation, deionization, and/or reverse osmosis techniques. Aquafina, bottled by Pepsi, is UV-disinfected and ozonated. On the other hand, Dasani, bottled and distributed by Coca-Cola, is treated with reverse osmosis filtration prior to bottling.

Unfortunately, even though one would think that bottled water is free from hazardous toxins and bacteria, the Environmental Working Group in 2009 revealed thirty-eight low-level contaminants in bottled water, including:

1. Disinfection byproducts
2. Caffeine
3. Tylenol
4. Nitrates
5. Industrial chemicals
6. Arsenic
7. Fluoride
8. Bacteria

Included within the broad group of "industrial chemicals" are contaminants associated with the storage and distribution of water in plastic bottles. Although approved by the FDA, chemicals found in plastics previously deemed safe for the handling and storage of food have been discovered to cause disease. These include:

- PBDEs (polybrominated diphenyl ethers) – Flame-retardant chemicals used in plastics. This category of chemicals has been linked to reproductive problems and thyroid disease.[22,23]
- Phthalates – Found in many household products, these are a family of chemicals that increase the flexibility of plastic, but are now known to disrupt the endocrine system. They have also been shown to damage the reproductive system in animals.[24]

- BPA (bisphenol A) – Another additive to plastic that has been shown to disrupt the endocrine system by mimicking the female hormone estrogen.[25,26] BPA is associated with unwanted hormonal effects in children and adults, even at low concentrations.[27] As a result, industry has largely replaced BPA. Unfortunately, "BPA-free" plastic containers have also been found to contain other estrogen-mimicking chemicals.[28]

There are numerous compounds used in the production of plastic and manufacturers are creating new chemical compounds each year. The potential for adverse health effects from many of them has yet to be determined.

If you do drink water from plastic containers, keep your plastic water bottles out of direct sunlight and away from all sources of heat, as heat increases the amount of chemicals that leaches out of the plastic and into the water. In addition, changes in pH can cause the chemicals in a plastic water bottle to leach into the water, so don't add a squirt of lemon juice, apple cider vinegar, or the like to your water.[29] Keep bottles away from detergents, cleansers, solvents, and automotive supplies and make sure that you don't handle your plastic water bottle if you have solvents such as paint thinners, gasoline, or other petroleum products, including Vaseline, on your hand, as they can be absorbed into the plastic. Even particles from solvents, including household cleaning products, if left uncapped, can aerosolize, attach, and become absorbed into plastic bottles, thereby diffusing into your water. Plastic bottles should not be washed in a dishwasher or by hand for reuse.

Reverse osmosis water provided by a manufacturer may initially be a more purified product than well water obtained from some locales, but after packaging and storage, it's hard to know exactly how safe any bottled water truly is. If you need to drink bottled water, opt for glass bottles whenever possible. Perrier is a good option if you like sparkling water. My suggestion, though, would be to have a home filter that will purify your well or tap water and then transport your drinking water with you in a reusable glass bottle for your daily use. Yes, it means that you have to plan ahead each day by filling your water bottle before you leave your house to go to school or work. It also means that you have to wash your glass bottle daily.

But think of all the money you will save by not buying bottled water every day. Not only that, you will be drinking healthier water and lessening your ecological footprint. Try it!

Purification

Whether you are getting your water supply from a public water system or a well, once the water is in your house, it should be purified. The specific purification method you choose will depend on your water source, what your level of contamination is, and your budget allowance.

There are several different purifying systems available for home use. These include gravity drip filters, ion exchange systems, and reverse osmosis systems. Not all water filters are created equal, and be aware that filters are not subjected to any governmental oversight or regulation. There is, however, the National Sanitation Foundation (NSF) international certification program, which provides certification and standards for many filters and can be reviewed when deciding which filter to purchase for your home.

Gravity systems use the weight of a column of water to push the water through a filter that removes contaminants. The main component of a gravity drip system is activated charcoal. Activated charcoal is a processed piece of carbon that has been treated with steam at high temperature, thereby making it porous, with millions of tiny air pockets. In this way, the surface area of the charcoal is increased dramatically, similar to the method your body uses for gas exchange (oxygen and carbon dioxide) in your lungs. Water and gases permeate through the charcoal, and as they do, contaminants attach to the charcoal and stay behind. Activated charcoal is excellent for removing many organic compounds, including VOCs, pesticides, herbicides, heavy metals, chlorine and its byproducts, bromine, and iodine. However, some inorganic ions, such as fluoride, sodium, and nitrates, and some organic compounds, such as acetone, methyl chloride, 1,4-dioxane, and isopropyl alcohol, do not adhere to charcoal and will not be removed by an activated charcoal filter.

The ability of activated charcoal to absorb chemicals is described in probabilities, as the efficiency of filtration and absorption is dependent on many different variables, including the temperature and pH of the water. As these decrease, absorption increases.[30] So a charcoal filter will remove the most contaminants from cold, acidic water.

Carbon filters need to be replaced periodically because as the binding sites get filled up a filter becomes less efficient, until finally, it no longer functions. The frequency for filter changes depends on how much water you drip through the filter and also on the porosity, or micron range, of the filter. Water will drip through a filter designed to remove tiny particles, down to 0.5 microns, slower than it will for a filter designed to remove particles measuring 5 microns or more, for example. A filter designed to remove tiny particles will also fill up with impurities faster and will need to be replaced more frequently. The micron range varies among systems and therefore the filters' efficiencies vary. Most cartridges designed to remove chlorine and eliminate odors and bad tastes are 10-micron cartridges.

The most inexpensive gravity drip filtration systems would include the canister systems widely distributed by Britta, Pur, etc. These companies also sell faucet attachments, which are similar in technology and remove a similar number of contaminants.

There are significant differences between vendors in the quality of contaminant removal. In 2014, a study by the Natural News Forensic Food Lab found that the company Zero Water made the gravity drip filter that provided the most significant removal of heavy metals. The more popular brands were found to be much less effective.[31] Bear in mind that these filters do not remove pathogens and should only be used with sterile or sanitized water.

More sophisticated gravity systems typically consist of at least two filters in series, one of which is usually an activated charcoal filter. The initial barrier in a more advanced gravity drip system may be a ceramic filter or micro-sponge that will limit the passage of particles into the rest of the filtration assembly. More common ceramic filters will optimally block all particles larger than two microns in size, thus eliminating almost all bacteria and microorganisms, including yeasts. Viruses, however, are smaller than two microns and will easily pass through many ceramic filters.[32]

Countertop gravity drip systems need to be refilled often, as the canisters that hold the treated water tend to be small. This is by design, so treated water does not stagnate and create the possibility of pathogens growing in the fresh filtered water.

Ion exchange systems are mainly used to deionize water or to soften water. Both types of systems work by passing water through different resins that exchange ions with the water. In deionized water all of the salts, including sodium, are removed. By contrast, softened water is processed to remove ions such as calcium, magnesium, and other metals from the water, while leaving behind sodium. The resulting water may taste salty, but it does not damage appliances, sinks, or faucets with the deposits common to hard water. Soft water also requires less soap for washing clothes or dishes and leaves less of a film on dishes and bathroom surfaces after washing.

The states with the hardest water sources are Florida, New Mexico, Arizona, Utah, Wyoming, Nebraska, South Dakota, Iowa, Wisconsin, and Indiana. Although deionizing and softening systems are very efficient at removing inorganic contaminants, they do not remove organic contaminants. If not maintained properly, these systems can become breeding grounds for bacteria. Ion exchange systems should be used in combination with a gravity drip system or a reverse osmosis system to remove organic contaminants and bacteria.

Reverse osmosis systems

The movement of water from an area with a lower concentration of salts (hypotonic) to an area of higher concentration of solutes (hypertonic) across a semipermeable membrane is known as osmosis. This natural phenomenon occurs until there is an equal concentration of solutes on either side of the membrane, a state referred to as equilibrium.

If, however, external pressure is exerted on a hypertonic solution, water flow in the opposite direction can occur. In this way, water is forced under pressure across the membrane from a hypertonic solution to a lower concentration of solutes. During this process, salts and other inorganic contaminants are held back by the membrane and are effectively removed from the water. This is the basis for the reverse osmosis (RO) water purification method. RO systems are excellent at removing inorganic contaminants, including ions, ethanol, and fluoride. This is a purification method that can even be used to desalinate sea water.[33]

RO water purifiers are usually placed in series with other filtration methods, similar to ion exchange systems. Most RO systems contain one or more activated carbon filters that remove chlorine and organic contaminants before the water hits the RO portion of the purification process. These "thin-film" RO units are the most common type sold. As RO systems have been shown to be breeding grounds for bacteria,[34] inline micropore filtration and UV systems are good ways to ensure that water coming from RO systems is safe to drink.

UV water purification

UV sterilization systems are commonly used in households that obtain water from private wells, particularly if the home relies on an ion exchange or RO filtration system. UV sterilization kills bacteria by denaturing their DNA with ultraviolet radiation, and has the advantage of being chemical free. As no chlorine is utilized, no chlorine byproducts are generated. UV systems are effective against *Cryptosporidium*[35], unlike the concentrations of chlorine typically used for routine sanitation. Although Giardia may be damaged by UV systems, it can sometimes still cause disease after treatment.[36] It is important to pass the water through a pre-filter before it is exposed to the UV light so that all sediment in the water will be removed. Sediment can provide an effective blockade for bacteria to hide behind as they pass through the UV rays. UV systems are not filters and do not remove any organic or inorganic contaminants.

Distillation

Only distillation is capable of removing virtually all of the contaminants found in water, including bacteria, inorganic salts, heavy metals, organic chemicals, and radioactive particles, but it is impractical for general home use. Distilling is also time-consuming and very expensive, because it requires a large amount of energy to produce a small amount of purified water. Demineralized water and distilled water in particular are not optimal sources of hydration for the body, as they are devoid of nutrients and needed minerals.[37]

Whole-house systems

A purification system designed to treat all of the water entering and distributed throughout a house is referred to as a whole-house system. All water purification methods offer whole-house systems. If you get water from a private well, it may make more sense to invest in a whole-house system than if you have access to a reliable public water supply. Technologies can be combined to ensure that you are not only removing organic and inorganic contaminants, but also bacteria. Ion exchange softening systems may be a worthwhile investment regardless of your water source, since they remove metals and therefore reduce water deposits, improving the life and performance of appliances. Water softeners also reduce the amount of soap needed for personal hygiene, laundry, and dishes. While external gravity drip systems are impractical for the whole house, they are useful at select faucets. Many companies make inline shower head filters, which remove chlorine and chloramine products before the water sprays onto your body. I highly recommend using one, especially if you are on a public water source or if your home system uses chlorine to disinfect your water.

All water treatment system companies should provide you with a performance data sheet that lists all the contaminants a system is certified to remove. Hundreds of companies make and/or distribute water purification systems and it would be unwise to purchase a product that does not supply a performance data sheet.

Once your water is purified, keep it stored in the refrigerator in a capped glass bottle. Bacteria could potentially grow in your purified water, so it must be consumed within a few weeks. The amount of water you consume will vary depending on your activity level and, of course, your physical size. If your urine is dark in color or is odiferous, then you aren't drinking enough water.

As you drink water, consider that it has a hidden, underlying organizational structure, as it is composed of billions of tiny magnets. Pure water will form a hexagonal shape when frozen and crystallized, akin to a snowflake. Masaru Emoto, a Japanese researcher, performed experiments that show focused attention to water will actually affect the energy flow within it and change the shape of the water crystals. Negative thoughts, such as anger and hate, had a disorganizing effect on the water's energy and inhibited crystallization. Although his scientific method was questioned and his findings were not published in the scientific literature, his work suggests that water will resonate with your intent as you focus upon it. If you bless the water by imparting positive feelings such as gratitude, love, or joy, in effect "praying" to the water, you will impart harmonious frequencies into the water, which you can then drink. Playing music will also affect the energy flow and vibrational frequency of water. I mindfully drink water and believe it does make a difference for my well-being. Provide "blessed" water to your pets and plants too, and take notice to see if there is any observable change in their health.

Researchers are beginning to prove that water can hold onto an electromagnetic frequency, which can cause biological effects.[38] A Japanese company, Nikken, has created a series of water filtration units that take into account the magnetic character of water. Their multistep filtration systems ultimately provide a magnetic filtration which is designed to cleanse the water of energetic impurities. The Nikken system produces water that then bathes in mineral rocks, creating a wonderful, slightly alkaline, mineral-rich

water, simulating river water. This system has been my choice
for water filtration for many years.

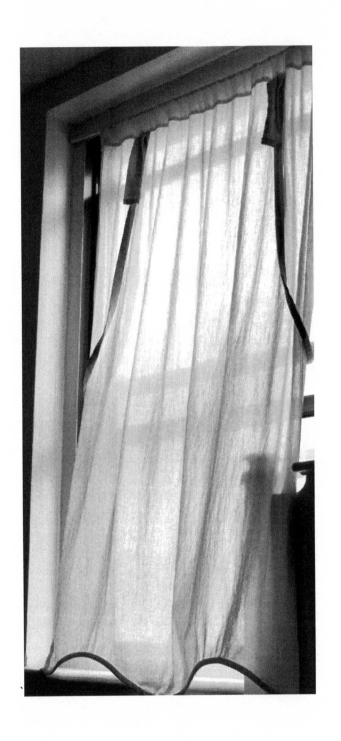

Chapter 2

AIR

Clean air is colorless, transparent, and intangible, yet it can contain all kinds of pollutants that make you sick. Some contaminants you can see with your eyes; others are invisible.

Air interacts with the body via two main mechanisms. You inhale air into your lungs during respiration (breathing) and you contact air with exposed surfaces of skin and mucous membranes. Breath is essential to life, but what exactly are we doing when we breathe? The body performs two functions with breath. One is to extract oxygen from the air because our cells utilize oxygen to produce energy and carry out their functions. The other is to release carbon dioxide, one of our body's waste products. The aggregation of oxygen from the air and the release of carbon dioxide from the body occurs in the lungs.

When we inhale, muscles in the chest wall expand and a large flat muscle that separates the chest cavity from the abdominal cavity, called the diaphragm, contracts, creating negative pressure in the chest. This results in the movement of air through the nose or mouth, down the windpipe (trachea), and then into the lungs through passageways called bronchi and bronchioles. These passageways split and divide many times, normally becoming narrower as they reach farther and farther into the lungs. At the end of each passageway, there is a little balloon-type structure called an alveolus. Tiny blood vessels called capillaries pass through the walls of the alveolus, and as the blood within them enters, a protein in the blood cell called hemoglobin releases the carbon dioxide in exchange for oxygen. The blood cells then move back to the heart, which pumps them throughout the body, providing needed oxygen.

This mechanism works because both oxygen and carbon dioxide form a reversible bond with hemoglobin.

When you exhale, the diaphragm and muscles of your chest relax and positive pressure is then exerted on your chest cavity. This causes air to flow backwards, out of the alveoli and through the bronchioles, bronchi, trachea, and finally out of your nose or mouth. This is the basic mechanism of respiration.

The body is well adapted—in most people—to clear out inhaled particulate debris. The cells that line the airways secrete mucous, which traps debris. Tiny hairs called cilia, which protrude from these cells, wave back and forth, moving the mucous and trapped debris up and out of the airway and into the back of the throat, where it is either swallowed or blown out of the nose during a sneeze. This mechanism helps keep the airways clean.

The other way in which we interact with air is via the skin, the largest organ of the body. Intact skin is lined by a layer of stratified squamous epithelium, which is the technical term to describe the layer of dead cells that forms a protective covering over the live cells. This layer of dead cells helps to prevent the underlying live skin cells from being harmed by the environment. Penetrating injuries, scrapes, and cuts cause a violation of this barrier and allow the environment to access the interior of the body. It has been shown that the outermost layers of skin absorb oxygen directly from the air.[1] For this reason, it is sometimes preferable to leave skin injuries uncovered and exposed to the air.

All cells in the body, including skin cells and the cells that line mucous membranes, are surrounded by a protective envelope of fatty molecules called phospholipids, referred to as the cell membrane. Aerosolized solvents that dissolve into fat are able to penetrate cell membranes and enter cells directly.

Gas exchange

We need to breathe air that has an adequate percentage of oxygen. In the atmosphere, air is composed of approximately 21% oxygen and 78% nitrogen. Carbon dioxide, water vapor, and other miscellaneous gases make up the remainder.

Indoor air is quite different, and the percentages of oxygen and other gases can vary dramatically, as many products in the home can emit gases and particulates that "pollute" the air.[2] When we breath polluted air, some health effects can be felt immediately (acute) while others occur over the long term (chronic). The physical effects of air pollution may depend on the specific type of pollutant, its concentration, and an individual's propensity for disease or underlying immune status. For instance, a similar dose of pollen or cat dander may not have any effect on one person, while for another, it may cause a hypersensitivity immune response.

Acute health effects from indoor air pollution can include irritation of the mucous membranes, particularly in the eyes, nose, and throat. Indoor air pollution can carry allergens, thereby increasing the occurrence of allergic reactions and asthmatic exacerbations.[3] Headaches, dizziness, fatigue, and fever are some additional generalized symptoms that may develop following exposure to some indoor air pollutants.[4]

Chronic exposure to indoor air pollutants is more insidious and includes various lung diseases, heart disease, and cancer.[5] The exact concentration of a pollutant, such as benzene, and the duration of exposure needed to cause chronic disease are not clearly defined. A healthy immune system can help prevent the development of chronic disease, but a weak immune system may be ineffective at preventing the chronic adverse health effects from ongoing exposure to air pollution. With this in mind, for your own health and the health of others living in or visiting your home, it is best to reduce the concentration of your indoor air pollutants as much as possible.

Asthma is a chronic health condition in which the lungs' airways become hypersensitive to chronic, repeated exposure of pollutants and other "triggers" that cause an allergic response. Triggers cause a transient narrowing or tightening down of the airways, reducing the flow of air into the lungs. If the airways are given a chance to relax for a prolonged period of time without irritation, the hypersensitivity response can lessen and even go away on its own.

Indoor air pollutants

The most common sources for air pollution in the home include the burning of combustible materials, which creates particulates, and gaseous emanations from building materials and products brought into the home for cleaning, grooming, and hobbies. Outdoor contaminants, including radon, pesticides, and outdoor air pollution, may also enter the home.

Most combustible materials release nitrogen dioxide (NO_2) and soot into the air. Heating systems, fireplaces, stoves, candles, and tobacco are all combustibles. NO_2 is an odorless and colorless gas that can irritate the eyes and nose and cause shortness of breath. Soot, which is floating particulates in the air, can be inhaled into the lungs, become lodged, and cause irritation and tissue damage. With sporadic exposure, trapped particulates can slowly be cleared. If, however, soot exposure is frequent, the particulates will not be effectively removed. The resulting irritation to the lungs' airways can lead to infections and diseases such as bronchitis, emphysema, and lung cancer. Radon, if present in the home's air, may attach to soot particulates and be inhaled into the lungs, where it can become stuck and potentially cause cancer.[6]

Combustible materials also emit carbon monoxide, an odorless and colorless gas that is particularly dangerous. At lower concentrations, carbon monoxide can cause vague, flu-like symptoms, such as dizziness, headaches, nausea, and fatigue.[7] At higher concentrations, however, carbon monoxide poisoning can cause death.[8] When inhaled, carbon monoxide enters the lungs and passes into the bloodstream where it binds to hemoglobin in the red blood cells. Unlike oxygen and carbon dioxide, carbon monoxide forms a permanent bond with the hemoglobin molecule. The affected blood cell becomes permanently damaged and unable to deliver oxygen to the rest of the body. Carbon monoxide effectively causes suffocation. It is important to install carbon monoxide detectors on each floor of your home and to keep batteries properly charged.

Candles

I first discovered the hidden danger of candles after bringing home a new pet bird, a cockatoo. One of the instructions given to us, as new bird owners, was not to burn candles in the same room as the bird. I didn't understand why burning a candle could be so dangerous for a bird. I enjoy the mood created by candles, but I've learned that there are many different types of candles on the market, some more toxic than others.

Candles may be paraffin-based or composed of beeswax or soy/ vegetable wax. Paraffin-based candles are most common and are typically the least expensive. Paraffin is a petroleum-based product. Burning paraffin candles in your home can release harmful dioxins and acrolein,[9] a compound also found in cigarette smoke that has been shown to cause lung cancer.[10] Paraffin candles have also been shown to be a major producer of indoor micro particulates, known as PM2.5 particles.[11] These can be inhaled deep into the lungs and difficult to eliminate.

Be wary of candles that utilize a metal cone for a wick. These cones may be made of lead, a lead alloy, or zinc. As the burning wick heats up the cone, lead can be emitted into the air.[12] These cones have been banned in the US by the Consumer Product Safety Commission (CPSC) since 2004, but they are still sold in other countries. The aerosolized lead released from these cones can coat the walls, flooring, and furniture in your home. Children who crawl or touch the walls and then put their hands, which may have lead residue on them, into their mouths are at particular risk for lead toxicity.

"Slow burning" candles, artificially scented candles, and incense should also be avoided as they may emit additional chemical pollutants such as acetaldehyde and benzene into your home.[13,14] Unfortunately, there are no reliable labels to separate real aromatherapy products from the synthetic competition. The cost of a candle does not indicate the quality of the product. Many high-end stores sell paraffin-based candles with synthetic fragrances.

Avoid paraffin candles, and instead invest in either beeswax or soy candles, which emit fewer harmful emissions.[15] According to current labeling laws, candles that are 49% paraffin and 51% beeswax may be labeled beeswax candles, so be aware that if you purchase a beeswax or soy candle, the label should specify 100% soy/vegetable wax or 100% beeswax.

Following a few simple tips will help to reduce indoor air pollution caused by candles. Keep your candle wicks trimmed and avoid burning candles in a drafty space. In addition, use a candle snuffer to extinguish the flame instead of blowing the candle out. With these simple modifications you can significantly reduce the amount of soot.

Reducing indoor soot

In order to minimize air pollutants from other combustible material in your home, there are a few things you can do. First, make sure that your furnace and hot water heater are properly vented, especially if they are powered by gas. Have your equipment inspected and serviced regularly. Always turn on the range hood exhaust fan when using a stovetop or oven, especially if you are using a gas stove. Importantly, make sure the exhaust is directed via ductwork to the outside. It is ironic, but while writing this chapter I discovered that the exhaust fan over my gas range was directed to a dead space above the kitchen cabinets, and not to the outside! Instead of ridding the house of the gases from the stove and oven, they were being dispersed throughout the house.

If you use a fireplace or burn wood for heat, make sure to open the flue. Have your furnace flue and chimney inspected and cleaned annually. If you use a wood stove, make sure the stove meets EPA standards and that the doors fit tightly on the unit.

If in an emergency situation you find yourself using a generator for energy, don't operate it in the house, no matter how cold it is outside. Generators should be placed as far away as possible from open windows, vents, and doors so the fumes don't waft into the house.

Smoking cigarettes, cigars, or pipes causes the release of numerous pollutants into the air. The effects of second-hand smoke are well documented.[16] Vaping an e-cigarette is marketed as a safer alternative to cigarettes, but who really knows? The chemicals that make up e-liquids are proprietary information and manufacturers are not required to label them or disclose the ingredients. Vaping fluids are reported to contain fewer chemicals than cigarettes, but it has been shown that vaping releases propylene glycol as well as other toxic chemicals into the air.[17] Some studies have shown that the "flavors" added to vaping fluid have been discovered to add toxic effects to e-cigarettes, with the most significant health effects attributed to the strawberry flavor.[18] Incredibly, these flavors have not yet undergone extensive testing.

Building materials and household products

The most common airborne pollutants associated with building material include asbestos, lead, and VOCs. Many people don't realize that asbestos is a naturally occurring mineral fiber that exists in rock and soil. Because of its strength and its high resistance to heat, it has been used in a variety of building materials for insulation and as a fire retardant. When it is disturbed by cutting, sanding, or drilling, the fibers can become transiently airborne and inhaled. These tiny needle-like fibrils get trapped in the lungs, where they cause inflammation. The cilia and mucous in the lung are unable to clear away the fibrils. Chronic exposure can lead to asbestosis, a disease characterized by lung scarring. The lining of the lung (the pleura) develops sheet-like regions of calcification, called pleural plaques, characteristic of asbestos-related disease. The lung and pleura both become at risk for cancer in the forms of lung carcinoma and mesothelioma. If you suspect there are products containing asbestos in your home, have them inspected and removed by a trained contractor. Under no circumstance should you attempt to remove asbestos yourself, unless you are certified to do so.

Lead was used for many years in the production of paint. When lead paint deteriorates or is removed improperly, the lead dust created can then be inhaled or ingested. Lead toxicity can damage the brain, spinal cord, kidneys, and blood cells. If children are exposed to lead, they can suffer physical and mental delays as well as behavioral problems.[20] As mentioned earlier, lead can also be emitted by some candles. If your home was built before 1978 and there is original paint on the walls, even if the paint is beneath wallpaper, don't remove the paint until you have it tested for lead. If the paint does contain lead, hire a trained professional to remove the paint. If the paint is in good condition, don't worry about the lead until it begins to deteriorate or until you want to remove it. If you or your partner work in an industry with lead products, make sure dusty clothes arechangedbeforeenteringthehome. Wash lead-tainted clothes separately from all other laundry. If your occupation exposes you to lead, eating a diet rich in calcium, phosphorus, and iron will help reduce lead absorption.[21,22]

Most of us are continually exposed to VOCs that emanate from building materials in the home. Any carbon-containing compound that exists as a gas at room temperature is a VOC. There are thousands of VOCs used in the production of building materials and pretty much any other fabricated item you might buy, some of which are listed in Table 2. Many VOCs are innocuous, but others are known carcinogens.

Table 2. Household consumer products containing VOCs

Paints and lacquers
Paint strippers
Paper towels
Carbonless copy paper
Grocery bags
Pesticides
Copier and printer inks
Permanent markers
Correction fluids
Cleaning supplies, including dish detergents and fabric softeners
Building furnishings, including carpets and vinyl flooring
Craft materials, including glues and adhesive
Clothing and dry-cleaning materials

Formaldehyde, one of the most common VOCs, is colorless, with a strong odor. It is used in the resins that make up composite wood products, including hardwood plywood, particleboard, and medium- density fiberboard. Although the emission of formaldehyde from building materials has been decreasing, formaldehyde concentrations in ambient indoor air have been continuously increasing.[23] This is likely due to its ubiquitous presence in household products.

Health consequences of formaldehyde depend on the duration of exposure and the concentration of the gas. Acute exposure can cause irritation of the eyes, coughing, and nausea, while chronic exposure has been associated with cancer, particularly nasopharyngeal carcinoma (throat cancer).[24] As with all VOCs, formaldehyde is a gas at room temperature, and slowly emanates from the products it is mixed into over time, a process referred to as off-gassing. As the air temperature or humidity in the house increases, the rate of off-gassing accelerates.

Although the EPA has set regulations to limit the concentration of formaldehyde in each product, there is no way to control the total amount of formaldehyde a homeowner may be exposed to. Indoor concentrations can rise to unhealthy levels when windows are closed and the heat is turned on. Mobile homes have been shown to off-gas particularly high levels of formaldehyde, especially in the wintertime.[25]

Other common VOCs found in building materials and household goods include methylene chloride, xylene, toluene, and benzene. Like formaldehyde, benzene is a known carcinogen which can damage the bone marrow and cause leukemia.[26]

All materials containing VOCs off-gas continuously. That luxurious new carpet you may have recently purchased is off-gassing, as is the new cabinetry in your kitchen and the fresh new paint applied to your walls. To drive home this point, I'd like to share a quick personal story.

A year ago, I decided to paint my living room with a faux plastering technique I had seen advertised at a local paint store. I purchased the needed supplies and went to work. The base coat went on smoothly, but the plastering layer required a more laborious technique of smearing arcs of dyed plaster material to the freshly painted wall. The instructions said to use the product in a well- ventilated area, so I left the overhead fan on continuously and the windows wide open. The process took me three days to complete, and at the end of the third day, I developed a nosebleed. This was unusual for me, as it was the middle of spring and I had only experienced nosebleeds in the winter when the air is dry for prolonged periods of time. The bleeding stopped without too much effort, but that night, I was awakened by another nosebleed. I applied pressure and it eventually stopped. Over the next two days, I experienced nosebleeds that became progressively more severe, coming out of not only one, but both nostrils simultaneously. I ended up at the emergency room of a local hospital where the staff packed my nose to stop the bleeding. Following this, the physician looked up both nostrils with a scope. He didn't see much but irritation. He blindly cauterized several areas in the back of my nose and sent me home, prescribing a follow-up appointment with an ear, nose, and throat specialist. I told him that I had just painted a room in my house, but he looked at me skeptically, as if I had given him a piece of history with no relevance. This ER physician, like most doctors, had no idea about the damaging effect that VOCs can have on nasal mucosa. The nosebleeds subsided after a few days and I have not had another one since.

A nosebleed is one physiological effect you can experience from the inhalation of VOCs. Many others are less obvious but can be much more dangerous.

If you are going to use a product such as a paint, plaster, adhesive, or solvent in your home, make sure to use the product in a well-ventilated area. This means to preferably use these products outdoors or in areas with an exhaust fan to the outdoors. If the product needs to be used indoors, as was the case with my paint, open up as many windows as possible and place a large fan in the room to provide as much outdoor air infiltration as possible. Off-gassing will continue for some time after a product has been applied and continued air ventilation is needed for at least a couple of weeks until the VOC levels have dropped sufficiently. Given the different chemicals in each brand of paint and the differing ambient conditions in each individual room, it is impossible to recommend a specific time frame for this. I would recommend ventilating a newly painted room for two or three weeks after painting. In addition, try to purchase paint that is designed to emit a lower concentration of VOCs. Your paint supplier should be able to help guide you to the best brands.

Once you are finished using a product that contains VOCs, move the container outside or into the garage, as these containers continue to leak gases. Please do not put empty containers into a garbage pail in your home to sit until garbage day. Toxic and hazardous household wastes need to be discarded responsibly. Ask your local government for proper disposal procedures.

Miscellaneous VOCs

There are many other sources of VOCs in your home. The more you are aware of, the more you may be able to remove. These may be in your closets, laundry rooms, or bathrooms. Go around your home and sniff. If your sense of smell is functioning, you will find many of these items on your own.

Do you have a mothball closet or use mothballs to protect your clothes? We had one in our house when I was a kid and it was down in the basement, away from the commonly used living areas. Clothing moths can be very destructive. There are many ways to prevent and rid your home of clothing moths, but using moth balls is one of the least desirable. The chemical paradichlorobenzene is a common active ingredient in moth repellents and is known to cause cancer in animals, but human effects are unclear.[27] It has been suggested that this chemical may even be associated with the development and progression of multiple sclerosis.[28] Instead of a creating a mothball closet, use a cedar chest or build a cedar closet. Alternatively, clothing bags and air-tight containers will seal your clothing and protect it from moths. Pheromone traps are also available for the closet. These are different than the ones used for pantry moths – make sure you use the correct trap.

Dry cleaning will rid clothing of moth larvae and eggs and is a preferable method for cleaning many delicate fabrics. But among the chemicals used in the dry cleaning process is perchloroethylene, a potent VOC that has also been shown to cause tissue damage and cancer in animals.[29] Hodgkin's lymphoma has been associated with occupational exposure to trichloroethylene, a related compound.[30] If your clothing is damp or has a chemical smell when you pick it up from the dry cleaner, you should leave the clothing at the store and tell them that they need to completely dry the clothing before you will take it home. Damp clothes from the dry cleaner will off-gas and fill your bedroom closets with toxic gas.

Dryer sheets and scented detergents contain VOCs that temporarily adhere to your clothing. There are less toxic alternatives to these fragrant products. If you want to make your clothes static-free, place a pair of clean old sneakers or some other type of unscented "laundry ball" into the dryer to reduce static cling. You can also create lavender packs or other dryer bags filled with herbs and essential oils that can make your clothing smell fragrant without using synthetic VOCs.

The same chemical used in moth repellents, paradichlorobenzene, is also used in many air fresheners and deodorizers. If you use these products in your home, it would be a terrific goal if you could slowly wean yourself from them. Proper ventilation and household cleanliness will prevent most unpleasant odors in the home without the need for chemical air fresheners. As you take steps to reduce the particulates in your air and reduce your home's VOC concentration, you will find that most odors will dissipate. If you do still have an odor problem, you should go on a search for mold.

Mold

Mold is a category of plant life that includes mushrooms and other wonderful organisms that are used to make many types of food, including bread, cheeses, sausages, and some types of medicine, including penicillin. Molds and fungi are an extraordinarily important component of the soil and for the outdoors.

Mold usually only becomes a health concern when it colonizes indoors, creating a musty, unpleasant odor by secreting microbial volatile organic compounds (MVOCs). Depending on the extent of the colonization, removal may be as simple as wiping down the area colonized and removing any source of moisture, such as a leaky pipe, and by opening windows or using fans to increase ventilation. If you have a significant amount of mold growing in your home, cleanup can be tricky and may require the help of a professional. Ceiling tiles, upholstered furniture, and carpets that have become moldy may need to be thrown out and replaced, as mold can lie dormant for long periods of time if the environment becomes dry. The mold will then awaken when humidity levels again increase.

Some molds may at times produce harmful toxins, called mycotoxins.[31] One type of mold, referred to as toxic black mold, can grow in moist, dark places in your home, usually in an area where there has been a hidden water leak, such as inside a wall or under a floor. This mold has a greenish- black gelatinous appearance when wet, and dries to a black powder. If disturbed, this mold can release huge numbers of spores and mycotoxins throughout your home. Toxic black mold is thought to be very dangerous and has been associated with mental impairment, breathing problems, and damage to internal organs.[32] If you find it in your home, you need to hire a professional black mold removal service to eradicate it. The longer you are around mold, and in particular, toxic black mold, the greater the chance it can damage your health.[33]

Molds grow locally in areas where there is excessive moisture caused by a leak, but a much larger area of mold growth can occur in your home if the air is too humid. There are packets and buckets containing anhydrous materials that will absorb moisture from the air and can help decrease local humidity in a small area of excessive dampness. If you live in an environment where the outdoor humidity is high or if you have underground living spaces that are damp, a dehumidifier is the easiest way to remedy excessive moisture from the air. Indoor air humidity should ideally be between 30% and 50%. If humidity is too high, molds will grow on many, if not all, surfaces in the room, producing millions of tiny spores that will be released and will float through the air. If the spores land on damp areas, they will stick, grow, spread, and reproduce, creating yet more spores. Molds may produce allergens, irritants, and sometimes toxins that, when inhaled, can cause allergies. Reducing the number of mold spores in your home requires both removing the existing colonies of mold and eliminating sources of moisture. An exhaust fan or an open window will help reduce moisture in the bathroom during and after your shower. An open window in the kitchen will also help water vapor escape if you are boiling liquids or washing dishes. Another potential area of mold accumulation is the laundry room. Front-loading washing machines sometimes hold on to moisture and can become breeding grounds for mold that can then attach to your clothing. Keeping the washing machine door open after each wash will allow the interior to completely dry out in between washes.

It is impossible to completely remove mold from your home, as mold spores are ubiquitous. But eliminating excessive moisture in the home will significantly reduce the quantity of mold spores and toxins, improving your health and eliminating odors.

Indoor pollutants that migrate indoors

Many pollutants commonly found outdoors find their way into our homes either through cracks and crevices in our walls and foundation or by our inadvertently tracking them inside on our footwear while walking into the house. The most dangerous of these toxins is radon.

Radon

If you only take one suggestion from this chapter, my hope would be that you will have your home tested for radon gas. Exposure to and inhalation of radon gas is the number-one cause of lung cancer among nonsmokers.[34] In 2009, the World Health Organization (WHO) declared radon gas in homes to be a worldwide health risk.

Radon gas is odorless, tasteless, and invisible, and therefore cannot be sensed by your brain. Radon is dangerous because it is radioactive; it is produced by the slow decay of uranium found naturally in soil and water. Radon is found in outdoor air in very low levels—0.4 pCi/L (picocuries per liter)—but can infiltrate your home through foundation cracks and accumulate in the indoor air. The average radon concentration inside American homes has been estimated to be 1.3 pCi/L, but may be much higher. The EPA has designated 4 pCi/L as the acceptable upper limit for radon concentration of indoor air.[35]

Radon is breathed in with air and can wreak havoc on the cells that line the airways in your lung. As with many types of radiation, the development of cancer isn't dose dependent. Therefore, it is best to limit the amount of radon in your home as much as possible.

Every home, everywhere, should be tested for radon gas, particularly in the basement. For many home buyers, mortgage companies require a radon inspection before approving a mortgage. Radon tests can be performed as either short-term or long-term tests. Short-term tests range from 2 to 90 days whereas the long-term tests accumulate data for over 90 days. A long-term test will provide information regarding your home's year-round average radon level. A long-term test is ideal, but a short-term test should suffice. If radon levels in your home lie between 2 and 4 pCi/L or higher, a process called remediation will help reduce the radon concentration in your indoor air. A radon specialist can install venting in the affected areas of your home to allow the gas to diffuse back outside.

Pesticides

Pesticides can significantly degrade indoor air quality. Many of these products are specifically designed for the indoors, including insect killer for ants, termites, bees, and other insects, and rodent killer for mice and rats. Pesticide liquids and collars may be applied to your pets. Pesticides may also be inadvertently tracked into the home after you walk in your garden or on your lawn after the outdoor application of pesticides and/or herbicides. Both the active and inactive ingredients in pesticides can aerosolize in the home and contaminate the air.

Pesticide exposure can cause both acute and chronic health problems. Researchers have found acute toxicity to cause headaches, blurred vision, dizziness, muscle cramping, shortness of breath, and many other symptoms.[36] Chronic exposure can damage the liver, kidneys, and peripheral nerves. Sensory nerves have particularly been shown to be damaged by chronic exposure to pesticides.[37] Some pesticides are associated with causing cancer.[38]

By taking a few precautions, you can significantly reduce the indoor accumulation of pesticides. First of all, have your family and guests remove their footwear upon entering your home. Apply flea and tick solutions to pets outdoors. If you spray or have a pest company spray your indoors with pesticides, ventilate the area afterward as much as possible by opening the windows and running fans until the odors dissipate. Even "non-toxic" products that are pet friendly should be ventilated. Store unused product in the garage or some other protected outside space.

The severity of outdoor air pollution depends on your home's location. If you live in an area with bad outdoor pollution, opening up the windows and doors in your home can bring small particles and ground-level ozone from car exhaust, smoke, road dust, and factory emissions into the home. Pollen from plants can also contribute to particulate air pollution. Outdoor air pollution levels fluctuate with the weather, industry activity, and the season, worsening with higher air temperatures and air stagnation. A windy day will clean out pollutants and provide cleaner air, but outdoor air will begin to concentrate contaminants again once the wind abates. Bad outdoor air quality can cause a real hardship when trying to achieve optimal indoor air quality. One of the easiest ways to clean up your indoor air is to open the windows and allow cross ventilation, but if the outdoor air is contaminated, this can have the opposite effect.

Other particulates

Particulate pollution consists of a mixture of microscopic aerosolized solids and liquid droplets categorized by size. Large particles are classified as PM10. The smallest particles are designated PM2.5. PM10 particles will get stuck to the mucous that lines the larger bronchioles and bronchi and cause an allergic response and an exacerbation of symptoms in people with lung diseases, such as asthma, bronchitis, or emphysema.[39] In a person with a normal respiratory system, the particles are then either removed by the immune system's white blood cells or brought by cilia, which line the airway, to the back of the throat, where the particulates are swallowed or sneezed out of the nose.

The PM2.5 particles are 2.5 micrometers in diameter and smaller. They are so tiny that when they are inhaled, they travel all the way down into the lungs' alveoli, where they get stuck. Here the particles sit, become absorbed, and cause inflammation and disease. Many health studies have shown a significant association between exposure to fine particles and premature death from heart or lung disease. Acute exposure to PM2.5 particles can cause fatal cardiac arrhythmias and heart attacks.[40]

What can be done?

Although there is no way to entirely rid your home of particulates and VOCs, steps can be taken to lessen the concentration of both.

Air cleaners

Air-cleaning devices remove particles from the air. The easiest way to lower the concentration of particulates in your home is to vacuum and dust regularly. Air cleaners will remove suspended particulates while dusting will remove settled material that can become transiently airborne by shuffling papers, walking, etc. For those with chronic lung disease, such as asthma, a dose of dust that contains allergens can set off an asthmatic attack.

Air filters are the most common form of air cleaner. They may be placed inline with your home HVAC system, or on a free-standing air purifier unit where they remove particulates from the airstream passing through the filter. Air filters are rated according to a minimum efficiency reporting value (MERV) unit ranging from 1 to 20. The higher the rating, the smaller the particles that will be trapped by the air filter. The most commonly used air filters used in residential homes to fit inline with air conditioners and furnaces typically have a MERV value of 1 to 4. These filters protect the HVAC equipment from the buildup of unwanted materials on the surfaces of the system, but don't improve indoor air quality. Pleated filters with a MERV value between 5 and 16 will remove both small and large airborne particles. Filters with MERV values over 7 are increasingly effective at removing particulates. Filters with a MERV value between 14 and 16 are almost as efficient as HEPA filters at absorbing PM2.5 particles, but may require increased fan and motor capacities if they are used with your home HVAC.

A true high-efficiency particulate arrestance (HEPA) filter is designated with a MERV value over 17. These filters will effectively remove PM2.5 particulates from your indoor air, but are not normally installed in residential HVAC systems, as they require modifications to the air- handling system. HEPA filters are more commonly available as portable units that can be moved from room to room. If your home is drafty and is located in a region with significant outdoor air pollution, consider that PM2.5 particles are being brought into your home daily, and invest in a HEPA filter. Removing PM2.5 particles from your indoor air will improve your health and longevity.[41]

If you purchase a portable air cleaner, be aware that these machines are rated according to their clean air delivery rate (CADR), a measure of how much contaminant-free air is delivered in cubic feet per minute. Evaluating the CADR will help you determine what size room a given filter will function best in. Although portable units, especially those with HEPA filters, are effective at removing microparticles, most portable air cleaners are ineffective at removing large particles, such as pollen and dust mites, which settle quickly on surfaces. Vacuum cleaners fitted with HEPA filters will draw up both and trap microparticles, removing them from the environment.

Electronic air cleaners and ionizers use a different technology than air filters to remove airborne particulates. Air cleaners draw air through an ionization chamber in which particles accumulate a charge. The charged particles then aggregate on a series of oppositely charged flat plates called collectors. Similarly, ionizers emit charged ions into the air that adhere to airborne particles, giving them a charge. The charged particles attract each other and nearby surfaces, such as walls or furniture, and settle faster.

There is no standard measure to compare the effectiveness of electronic air filters. In general, ionizers and electronic air cleaners are not as effective at removing microparticles as filters are. In addition, they can create more indoor air pollutants by producing toxic ozone and ultra-fine particles (PM2.5) when reacting with VOCs from cleaning products, air fresheners, etc.[42] For these reasons, I would not recommend investing in an electronic air cleaner.

Ultraviolet germicidal irradiation (UVGI) cleaners use UV lamps to destroy viruses, bacteria, allergens, and molds, which are all pathogens that can grow on HVAC surfaces such as ductwork, drain pans, and cooling coils. UVGI cleaners need to be used in combination with a filtration system.

Unless you live in an area with poor outdoor air quality, an HVAC inline pleated air filter with a MERV value between 5 and 14 should suffice for particulate removal. Remember to change the filter at least once every six months. Consider purchasing a portable HEPA air filter and keep it running in your bedroom or whichever living space you spend most of your time in. If you or your child has asthma, this will further help keep down the level of PM2.5 particles in the treated room. In addition, by vacuuming and dusting the home at least once a week with a vacuum fitted with a HEPA filter, the concentration of dust in home air will significantly diminish. Make sure to steer away from HEPA filters that masquerade as synthetic air fresheners—these actually release VOCs into the air as you vacuum.

Tackling VOCs

To begin ridding your inside air of VOCs, first get in the habit of ventilating your home, especially during the winter months. In older construction, outdoor air flows into your home (infiltrates) through openings in the joints and through cracks in walls, floors, and ceilings and around windows and doors. Infiltration dilutes indoor air pollution by infusing fresh air.

Take care to strike a balance between not letting too much outdoor particulate pollution into the home and letting out the buildup of indoor VOCs. "Sick building syndrome" is a condition that has been attributed to spending long periods of time in buildings with construction techniques that use air-tight building envelopes to achieve energy efficiency. Since there is no exchange of air with the outside environment, indoor air pollutants build up and occupants become ill.[43] Regardless of the type of home construction you have, open the windows and turn on overhead fans frequently. Unless you live in an area with bad air pollution, chances are that the air outside is cleaner than the air inside, especially if you have had the doors and windows closed up for some time.

Next, you may want to try using portable air purifiers in rooms you spend the most time in. Many contain activated carbon pre-filters that help remove VOCs. An all-in-one portable air purifier contains a HEPA filter, a carbon filter, and a UV lamp to remove PM particles and VOCs to prevent the spread of bacteria and viruses.

Phytoremediation

My personal favorite solution for reducing indoor VOC concentration is to introduce houseplants. Growing indoor plants is an excellent, inexpensive method for removing VOCs from the indoor air through a process known as phytoremediation. Studies by many scientists, including those from NASA, Penn State University, the University of Georgia, and other institutions, have shown that plants can absorb a long list of VOCs, including benzene, toluene, xylene, and formaldehyde.[44,45] Once absorbed, bacteria on the plant roots convert the VOCs into nutrients for the plant. Most leafy plants can purify indoor air, and different plant species absorb different VOCs, so it is optimal to have several varieties within your home to cover all bases.[46] Many plants have proven to be effective at removing VOCs from inside air (Table 3).

Table 3. Common houseplants able to remove VOCs

crotons
spider plants
Schefflera plants
purple waffle plants
English ivy
golden pothos
Aloe vera
snake plants (mother-in-law's tongue)
peace lilies
corn plants
sentry palms

Choose a few plants to place in the kitchen, bedrooms, and living room. Take care of your plants as if they were pets. In return, they will protect you by producing oxygen and by absorbing VOCs from the air.

Optimizing your indoor air: negative ions

After you remove particulates and VOCs from the indoor air, you can optimize your air in several ways. The first is to create an atmosphere containing negative ions.

Negative ions were once studied for their physiological effects, but due to overreaching claims that they could cure everything, including cancer, they were lumped in with other types of voodoo medicine. Could this reputation have been created by industry? Possibly. Regardless, research has shown that negative ions can help to alleviate depression, reduce the stress response, and boost daytime energy, possibly by causing decreased responsiveness by the brain to serotonin.[47,48] Exposure to negative ions has been shown to decrease drowsiness, increase performance, and improve mental energy.[49,50,51] Seasonal affective disorder (SAD) has also been shown to respond to negative ion therapy.[52,53]

Negative ions are transient, for they lose their charge and become neutralized by forming chemical bonds with positive ions. Frequent or even continuous production of negative ions may be most desirable. Turning on the shower or bath will produce a large transient influx of negative ions into your bathroom, akin to a waterfall,[54] which may be why many of us love our morning showers. Opening the windows and allowing cross ventilation will also bring negative ions into the home.[55]

Ion generators can be installed into home HVAC systems, where they can be particularly restorative in the summer, since air conditioning systems deplete inside air of negative ions.[56] Some portable air cleaners contain negative ion-generating components.

Indoor plants generate negative ions as they are exposed to direct sunlight and undergo photosynthesis. Indoor water features with small cascades of flowing water may also generate negative ions and can be placed in living spaces.

Himalayan salt lamps are decorative elements that proponents say release negative ions when lit. These lamps come with either a depression to insert a beeswax candle or with a light bulb within. Although not scientifically validated, I have spoken with many people who say they find these salt lamps comforting and that they help to reduce anxiety and depressive symptoms. As with the other types of ion generation, the range of air affected by the salt lamp is limited, so if you consider trying one of these out, place the lamps in strategic locations where they will be most helpful.

Choose one or more of the above methods for generating negative ions in your bedroom and perhaps your living room. Use a negative ion generator before going to bed and while relaxing in your living room, particularly during those times of the year when your air conditioner is used or when your windows remain closed during the day. As negative ion generators do not create any aroma, you may find the addition of fragrance to your indoor air to be even more appealing.

Aromatherapy

Aromatherapy is not used to hide unpleasant odors. Rather, it is a form of alternative medicine that uses plant extracts and aromatic plant oils to alter one's mood and improve cognitive, psychological, and physical well- being.[57] By doing so, aromatherapy allows the body's immune system to strengthen and improves one's ability to heal. Aromatherapy has become a large field of study, with the goal of creating balance of the body, mind, and spirit.

Many companies capitalizing on the "fad" of aromatherapy have created synthetic fragrances and infused their oils and candles with them, instead of using genuine plant material. Chemists may tell you that the active ingredient in the synthetic variety is the same as in the plant extract, but those who use these products will tell you that the physiological effects are not the same.[58] Not only are the benefits of the aromatherapy reportedly lost in synthetic production, the synthetic varieties generate VOCs, which can degrade air quality instead of enhancing it![59]

Medical research on the effectiveness of aromatherapy is limited, but growing. These products are not regulated by the FDA, so if you decide to try out aromatherapy for your home, make sure you purchase genuine plant extract materials and essential oils. Aromatherapy oils can be placed on dryer balls, placed into diffusers, mixed with beeswax in candles, or dripped onto potpourri.

The Lampe Berger is a unique form of diffuser which has been around since 1898, when it was first created by a Parisian pharmacist named Maurice Berger. According to its manufacturer's website, this diffuser was initially conceived as a way to limit the spread of sepsis within hospitals by purifying the air. These products are not used in hospitals anymore but are mainly used in businesses and in homes, where they rid a room of undesirable odors and produce a subtle relaxing fragrance. I have enjoyed using a Lampe Berger for many years. Different fragrances can be used to create different moods in different rooms. These diffusers have not been found to produce benzene, styrene, naphthalene, formaldehyde, or acetaldehyde. They do produce some ozone, but at safe levels.

I'd recommend investigating aromatherapy. Choose an appealing fragrance and pick a method of dispersion. Try it and see how you feel with its use. With clean, optimized air, your home will truly become a refuge, a place to relax.

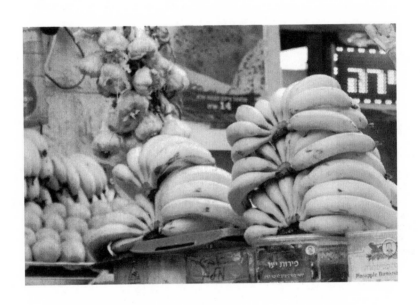

Chapter 3
WHOLE FOOD

Food. We eat it every day, but have you given any thought to why your body needs food? Yes, food can taste good, especially processed foods that have been designed to tweak your salt and sweet taste buds. (Do you think the flavor "salted caramel" is an accident?) But food has much more importance to us than the sensual pleasure of taste.

The food industry developed to feed people who were unable to grow their own food. As populations grew and more people moved to cities, the need to feed larger numbers of people increased. With increasing competition, food companies began to develop strategies to gain market share. Markets and supermarkets opened, providing all the food that had previously been purchased from individual vendors like the milkman, the farmer's market, the butcher, etc. The results of this evolution are delicious, visually appealing food products that last a very long time on store shelves. The industrialization and "perfection" of whole foods like fruits and vegetables has also occurred over time. The oversized, perfectly shaped, shiny bright apple is by human design, not by natural selection.

But as biological organisms who developed in a natural world, our digestive systems are adapted to eat foods in their natural state or processed through heat or fermentation, not by industrial chemistry. Organs such as the pancreas have evolved to produce specific proteins called enzymes, which are secreted into the intestine to help us digest the food we eat. Chemically altered food may or may not be able to be digested by this set of enzymes and instead may be evacuated partially digested or undigested. Synthetic chemicals can create havoc on the beneficial bacteria lining the system. In addition, depending on the integrity of the cells lining the tract, some of these manmade molecules may be absorbed into the bloodstream.

Anatomy/physiology

The system responsible for the internal processing of food is called the digestive system. The digestive system typically begins as food enters a long tube at an orifice in your face called a mouth. From there, food passes through many compartments, including the esophagus, stomach, small intestine, and large intestine. Waste material typically exits your body through the anus. Surgical techniques can alter this arrangement at any step along the way. The digestive tract is not pretty, but its basic function isn't too complicated to understand.

In your mouth, the mechanical process of chewing grinds and macerates food into smaller bits. While chewing, food is moistened with saliva, which not only softens the food, but also begins the digestion of starches. Your tongue, given the presence of numerous taste buds all along its surface, is able to provide sensation to your brain about the quality of the food in your mouth before you swallow it. Is it sweet? Sour? Salty? Bitter? A combination of these?

Once swallowed, the food travels through the esophagus and into the stomach, where it usually sits for several hours while it contracts and churns, mixing with acid and enzymes to begin the digestion of proteins. A muscular ring, called a sphincter, which separates the top of the stomach from the esophagus, is normally tightly closed during this process to prevent refluxing of the acids and food material back into the esophagus.

Once the food is sufficiently mashed up, the chyme, as it is now referred to, passes out of the stomach, a bit at a time, and into the first portion of the small intestine, called the duodenum. As this happens, two different fluids, bile and pancreatic juice, empty into the duodenum through a duct. Both fluids mix with the chyme to help further digest it. Bile emulsifies fats, breaking them down into their components, fatty acids and glycerol. The pancreatic enzymes work on breaking down proteins, fats, and starches into their building-block components. Lactase, the enzyme able to break down the milk protein lactose, is one of the pancreatic enzymes released.

The resulting mixture passes through many feet of small intestine, which provides plenty of time and surface area for the food materials to break down into their molecular components. Once these molecules are small enough, the resulting peptides (or amino acids), sugars, and fatty acids are able to pass through the lining of the small intestine and into a bloodstream that leads directly to the liver.

The liver is a very complex organ with hundreds of functions, but you can think of it as a gatekeeper that regulates the amounts of sugar, fat, and protein that are allowed to pass into the bloodstream. From the components it receives from the small intestine, the liver assembles various proteins, fats, and cholesterol. Along with the pancreas, the liver is also involved with carbohydrate metabolism, or the storage and release of sugars into the bloodstream. The liver also very importantly acts as a toxin waste dump for those materials that pass through the lining of our intestines but aren't supposed to gain access to the rest of our body. We can survive without portions of the liver, but our bodies cannot survive without some functioning liver tissue.

Materials that are not able to pass through the wall of the small intestine collect in the large intestine, also referred to as the colon. The large intestine has three main functions. One is to act like a sponge and absorb excess water so we don't dehydrate. When the colon is irritated and not functioning properly, it doesn't absorb as it should and we can end up with diarrhea. Billions of bacteria also live in the large intestine, making it a very important part of the microbiome (the individual collection of bacteria that lines our guts, airways, and skin). These bacteria consume the food residue that passes by, and in exchange provide us with important minerals and vitamins including vitamin K and biotin.[1] The third important function of the colon is to absorb these vitamins, which are important for good health. The colon creates a solid material from the undigested remainder, referred to as stool, which passes into the rectum, where it is stored in preparation for evacuation through the anus.

In summary, our digestive systems, by utilizing chemical and mechanical processes, enable our bodies to break down foods into their components, absorb the nutrients, and expel the waste. Nutrients from the food we eat are absorbed through the small intestine, and the large intestine absorbs water, along with the vitamins and minerals released by bacteria.

Our bodies are composed of trillions of cells which are continually performing their daily functions: making proteins, reproducing, and dying. Nutrients, including fatty acids, cholesterol, amino acids/peptides, sugars, vitamins, and minerals, are needed to create more DNA and the material to build more cells. Without the influx of nutrients, our cells cannot function or reproduce and will eventually die. With prolonged starvation, organs fail and eventually, the whole body will die. Dietary sugars, fats, and proteins are all important foodstuffs we need for normal metabolism.

The food industry

With the development of supermarkets and the food industry, the need for food preservation and prolonged shelf life became very important. The food industry has expended tremendous resources to develop techniques to make food more visually appealing and better tasting, including the hybridization of crops and the application of waxes and chemical sprays to prevent food from decaying. Why buy an apple with a bad spot if there are blemish-free apples next to it?

In most US supermarket chains, the store's perimeter will house the "whole" foods, including produce, meats, poultry, dairy, and eggs. The center of the typical grocery store is reserved for processed foods and canned goods. This chapter concentrates on the whole foods perimeter, and the next chapter will focus on processed foods.

Produce

Perhaps the section of the supermarket that has gotten the most attention from food activists in recent years is the first section you typically walk into, the produce section. One of the biggest concerns in eating fruits and vegetables from a "conventional" market is the residue of pesticides, fungicides, and herbicides applied during the growing process. Stabilizers and other processing techniques designed to improve shelf life and product appeal are also suspect.

Anyone who has tried to grow an organic garden or orchard will agree that fighting off Mother Nature's creatures is a full-time task that can be daunting. Considering the ubiquitous presence of insects, weeds, and fungal diseases, it is no wonder that commercial growers have relied on pesticides, herbicides, and fungicides in order to help produce healthy and sizable harvests. Without these chemical products, there would be a lot less fruit and vegetables for us all to eat.

There are hundreds, perhaps even thousands, of different types of chemicals on the market to help growers produce bountiful harvests. Some chemicals are considered organic, and others conventional, or nonorganic. Organic sprays are considered more ecologically responsible and safe, but both of these types of sprays need to be removed from the food before it is eaten. If the skin on the fruit's surface is porous, the chemicals will be absorbed into the cuticle.[2] For this reason, I prefer organic fruits and vegetables. Pesticide residues will adhere the most to fruits and vegetables that contain a soft skin or waxy surface and should be removed with the aid of a fruit and vegetable spray wash, as many pesticides are not water soluble.[3] Peeling the fruit will remove the greatest amount of pesticide residue.[4]

There is a helpful resource produced by the Environmental Working Group (EWG), a nonprofit environmental research organization (www. ewg.org), that categorizes produce into the varieties that contain the most and least pesticide residue during a given year. In 2017, the foods that contained the greatest number of pesticides in the highest concentration, also known as the "dirty dozen," included:

Apples	Peaches
Nectarines	Strawberries
Grapes	Celery
Spinach	Sweet bell peppers
Cherries	Tomatoes
Pears	Potatoes

The EWG found that nonorganic leafy greens, including kale, lettuce, and collard greens, as well as hot peppers, were frequently contaminated with insecticides toxic to the human nervous system and that only organic versions should be eaten.

In 2017, the foods that contained the least amount of pesticide residue included:

Onions	Avocado
Sweet corn	Grapefruit
Pineapple	Mango
Honeydew	Broccoli
Frozen sweet peas	Kiwi
Eggplant	Sweet potato
Cabbage	Papaya
Cantaloupe	Cauliflower

There have been many scientific studies linking pesticide exposure to all kinds of health problems, including hormonal and reproductive problems as well as many different kinds of cancer, particularly in children.[5,6] Several long-term observational studies have indicated that organophosphate insecticides may impair children's brain development.[7] In 2012, the American Academy of Pediatrics issued a report specifying that children have a "unique susceptibility to the toxic effects of pesticide residue."[8] Pesticides are damaging to our health and care should be taken avoid inadvertently ingesting them.

Genetically modified organisms (GMOs) present a unique problem in that the pesticides and herbicides in these vegetables cannot always be washed off. GMOs are typically grown in herbicide-laden soil, and may have their DNA engineered to produce their own pesticides, thereby killing any insects that try and eat them. Unfortunately for us, the same corn kernel or soy bean that we eat contains the pesticide internally, which cannot be washed off. These herbicide-containing and pesticide- producing plants, when eaten, may have negative health effects that we do not completely understand. There is concern that our microbiome can be severely damaged by ingesting pesticides. This may be causing a significant increase in digestive disorders, including obesity and diabetes.[9,10]

The GMO story began with the creation of a chemical called glyphosate by Stafford Chemical in 1960. This chemical was created to bind with metals and was used as a descaling agent to clean industrial pipes of mineral deposits. The chemical company Monsanto purchased the chemical in 1969 and re-patented it as a nonselective herbicide. Thus, Roundup was born. Any homeowner or lawn maintenance worker will tell you that it is a lot easier to spray a chemical such as Roundup on a plant to kill it than it is to manually remove the plant with its roots.

Monsanto subsequently spent many years in the field of biotechnology, creating seeds that could grow in the presence of glyphosate. The idea was that it would be convenient for growers (and hugely profitable for Monsanto) to kill all the weeds in a field with Roundup and then grow a crop on the treated soil without the need for weeding during the growing season. In 1996, Monsanto created soybean seeds and corn seeds that could do just that, known as Roundup-ready soybeans and Roundup- ready corn. Farmers could spray their fields with Roundup and then plant the Roundup-ready seeds for a productive and reliable harvest. This technology was incredibly successful. By 2014, most soy and corn grown around the country was genetically modified. In 2016, according to the USDA, 92% of corn and 94% of soybean crops planted in the US were genetically modified.[11] Since the advent of Roundup-ready soy and Roundup-ready corn, Monsanto and other companies such as Dow and Dupont have created further GMO varieties, including sugar beets, canola, squash, and Hawaiian papaya. GMO varieties of wheat have also been the subject of experimentation, along with many other types of vegetables.

Unfortunately, as research has slowly accumulated, we are discovering that this biotechnology is not without significant health costs to all who eat these foods, including our cattle, chickens, and pigs, as well as our dogs and cats. Although the USDA declared GMO foods to be substantially equivalent to their non-GMO counterparts, the nutritional value of GMO foods is not equal to non-GMO food. This is at least in part due to the chelating properties of glyphosate. Glyphosate has been found to cause mineral depletion in the GMO soybeans[12] and in other GMO plants.[13]

Furthermore, GMO plants grown in soil treated with glyphosate absorb the chemical, depositing it in the plant's cells.[14] This means that there are traces of glyphosate in the soybeans and corn kernels used to feed our livestock and to produce processed foods—in other words, in the entire industrial food supply.

Glyphosate is an herbicide and has been found to be an effective antibiotic. In fact, in 2010, Monsanto received a patent for Roundup to be considered an antibiotic at concentrations as low as 1-2 mg per kg of body weight.[15] But scientists have shown that glyphosate disrupts the microbiome.[16,17] Eating foods laced with Roundup therefore can affect our digestion by killing off intestinal bacteria that produce nutrients and vitamins but also by binding to nutrients, making them unusable.

Damaging the microbiome does more to your health than affect your digestion or cause some diarrhea. A damaged microbiome has been associated with a hypersensitive immune system, resulting in asthma and increased allergies.[18] The conclusion of some researchers is that celiac disease, also known as sprue, has little to do with gluten sensitivity, but more to do with a glyphosate-damaged microbiome.[19] Know anyone with celiac disease? Twenty years ago, it was extremely rare. Today, it is unfortunately very common.

Perhaps one of the most concerning properties of glyphosate is that it does not get expelled with stool. After eating a vegetable or other food that contains glyphosate, some glyphosate will be absorbed by the intestine, where it can damage the intestinal lining.[20] Glyphosate has been found in human urine and has been shown to bioaccumulate in the kidneys, liver, spleen, and muscles in animals.[21] Once absorbed, glyphosate has been shown to disrupt the endocrine system.[22] It has also been shown to induce breast cancer growth.[23] Studies have shown that higher levels of glyphosate residue have been found in the urine of chronically ill people. In fact, the EPA website states that people drinking water containing more than 0.7 ppm of glyphosate may develop kidney problems and infertility.

Although the EPA acknowledges glyphosate as a food contaminant and has established legal residue limits, the FDA has been criticized for failing to disclose that they don't test food for residues from glyphosate and many other commonly used pesticides.[24] In addition, maximum residue levels (MRLs) have increased considerably over the years in the US and in other countries utilizing GMO technology in order to accommodate the new reality that glyphosate residue is ubiquitous within the food supply.

Some researchers have concluded that the widespread usage of herbicides and pesticides has caused epidemics of inflammatory and degenerative diseases, as well as all kinds of cancer, autism, and obesity, which have developed over the past twenty years.[25] Although many types of environmental toxins have been on the rise, the manipulation of our food supply has most likely had profound effects on society's overall health.

Root vegetables

If you have been around a while, you may remember going to the market and seeing "eyes" in the potatoes that would sprout if the potatoes were left on the shelf for too long. For many years now, root vegetables such as onions, potatoes, and carrots have been sprayed during growth with an herbicide that functions as an anti-sprouting chemical, preventing the vegetable from continuing its life cycle after harvest. The chemical, typically chlorpropham or maleic hydrazide, prevents cellular division. Yes, this chemical can affect human cellular division, too.[26] And residues of this chemical have been found on potato samples and even in potato chips![27] Japan and the EU have placed strict limitations on the usage of anti-sprouting chemicals, but there are no regulations for their usage in the US. For this reason, it is best to buy organic root vegetables.

Consider though, that potato sprouts are poisonous and should never be eaten. In addition, potatoes that have been exposed to light will turn green due to the stimulation of chlorophyll formation. The green parts of a potato contain the greatest concentration of alkaloids such as solanine, which can cause many symptoms, including increased sensitivity, shortness of breath, and gastrointestinal symptoms such as abdominal pain, nausea, diarrhea, and vomiting in higher concentrations.[28] For this reason, keep your potatoes in a cool, dark place, cut out any green areas and remove sprouts before cooking and eating them.

Food dyes

As many commercially grown apples and other fruits are picked before they ripen and achieve optimal color, fruits are commonly dyed to make them more appealing. In many instances, there is no way to tell if a fruit has been dyed, although I do remember years back occasionally biting into apples and noticing red streaks extending into the pulp from the skin, an obvious indication of dye. Florida orange growers use Citrus Red #2 dye to make their oranges look richer in color off-season. California and Arizona have banned the use of this dye, so if you want to be sure that your oranges haven't been dyed, buy them from California or Arizona growers. Although the FDA banned Red Dye #2 for use in food because it was proven to be carcinogenic, this dye has been approved for use on oranges because it is assumed that people don't eat the peel. But what if you put an orange wedge in your drink or use the zest in a recipe?

Commercial dyes are often created from petrochemicals. Over the years, many artificial colors have been banned and pulled off the market because they were found to be toxic. But several artificial dyes that have been found to cause behavioral problems in children, and even be carcinogenic, remain in the market.[29] Interestingly, in Europe, most foods that contain any of six artificial dyes associated with behavioral problems must be labeled, "May have effects on activity and attention in children."[30]

Waxes

After the application of dye, fruit may be coated in a fine layer of wax or paraffin so that it won't decay as quickly on the store shelf. There are many types of wax that are considered food grade and safe to eat. Conventional produce manufacturers apply petroleum-based wax to the fruit while organic suppliers apply beeswax or other natural waxes such as carnauba wax or shellac. Regardless of which type of wax is applied, pesticide residues can adhere to the wax layer.[31]

Using a fruit and vegetable wash soap will help wash off the wax so that more of the pesticide can be removed. Dish soaps, bleach, and other potentially toxic cleaners should not be used when cleaning fruits and vegetables because they can become absorbed by the pores of the fruit and themselves become contaminants. Unfortunately, no method, not even peeling, is 100% effective for removing all pesticide residues.[32]

Wax is used most commonly in cucumbers, peppers, eggplants, potatoes, apples, lemons, oranges, and limes. All of these fruits and vegetables should be washed with a fruit and vegetable spray. If you garnish drinks with citrus wedges or cook with the zest or skins, be sure to wash these fruits too, regardless of whether or not they are organic.

Packaging gases

Prepackaged produce, such as containers of lettuce, are commonly sealed with nitrogen gas, rather than air. Without the ability to oxidize, the enclosed vegetable will take much longer to decay, thus improving shelf life. This is an effective and relatively harmless way to improve shelf life.[33]

Irradiation

Another process that can increase shelf life for food products is irradiation. Some types of foods are irradiated to eliminate microorganisms that can cause food-borne illness.[34] As one would expect, beneficial bacteria are also destroyed in the process. According to the FDA website though, irradiation of food does not do anything to compromise its nutritional quality nor does it change the taste, texture, or appearance. As a radiologist, however, I am well aware that ionizing radiation denatures proteins.

Labeling is required for food that has undergone this process. The first food to be approved for irradiation in the US was wheat flour, in 1963, to help control mold growth. Since then, potatoes, pork products, fruits, vegetables, herbs, poultry, and meats have been approved for irradiation. Below is the required symbol to indicate a food has been irradiated (Figure 2).

Figure 2. Required label for irradiated food

The meat department

Before the industrialization of food, cattle, pigs, sheep, and goats were pastured and slaughtered for their meat once they were physically mature, except in the case of veal and lamb. The amount of time needed for an animal to grow to sufficient size was dictated by the quality of the pasture, the weather, and the genetics of the breed.

The industrialization of meat brought us images of horrific living standards and inhumane slaughtering processes in factory farms. Instead of grazing on grasses, these cattle may be tied to posts in feed lots where they are fed grain, such as GMO corn.

In the US and in many other countries, hormones are administered to the livestock to make the animals grow faster. Many steroid hormone drugs, including natural estrogen, progesterone, testosterone, and their synthetic versions have been approved by the FDA for use in beef cattle and sheep. The EU has not given approval to these same drugs. The FDA has not approved steroid hormones for growth purposes in dairy cattle, veal calves, pigs, or poultry.

Animals in factory farms are commonly injected with antibiotics to help protect them from the increased risk of illness that comes from their dirty, confined living quarters and their unnatural food source. The FDA has approved prophylactic antibiotic use for animals until slaughter. It was only until recently that the FDA allowed the administration of arsenic to cattle—after detecting arsenic in meat, the FDA finally removed it from the list of acceptable treatments in 2015.[35] The widespread use of antibiotics has come under more scrutiny as superbugs, resistant to antibiotics, are becoming more and more common.

In addition to antibiotics and an unnatural diet, factory-farmed meat can also be altered by the animals' stress levels. Stress causes the excessive production of cortisol, which leads to biochemical changes in an animal's cells. Meat from a stressed animal will have a different color, tenderness, and perishability than the meat from a non-stressed animal.[36]

In a spiritual sense, when eating, one consumes a physical form with an underlying frequency and energy. Eating the meat of a healthy, vibrant animal may impart a greater sense of well-being to us than eating the meat from an animal that has been chained to a feed lot, living a life of constant stress. Respect for an animal's "energy" permeates many cultures around the world. I wonder if the energy within the meat might be even more important for our health and well-being than the biochemical makeup of the meat.

If you choose to eat beef, lamb, pork, and veal, it is best to eat organic varieties, or in the case of beef, grass-fed beef. A label from the American Grassfed Association will reliably indicate that you are purchasing grass-fed beef that has not been fed corn. Depending on where you live, local farmers may pasture their cattle without injecting them with steroids or antibiotics. You can have a quarter or side of beef sectioned into various cuts, and many packages of ground beef as well. This is not only economical, but you know that you are eating the meat from one cow.

The fish counter

Fish and seafood are an excellent source of protein and nutrition, but the world's oceans have become polluted with materials ranging from plastics to hard metals. Mercury is the third most toxic naturally occurring substance in the world, behind lead and arsenic.[37] Methyl mercury is the most toxic contaminant in the world's fish. Coal-fired power plants, which emit particulates into the air, including mercury, have rained toxins upon the world's oceans, elevating mercury levels in the fish that live there. Thankfully, these plants are slowly either being phased out or retrofitted with scrubbers that remove dangerous contaminants before exhaust is emitted into the air.

I taught my children about the mercury in fish early in their lives. During a beach vacation one summer, my family and some friends were waiting on a dock to embark on an evening cruise boat so we could enjoy the sunset on the water. Fishermen had come in from a day at sea and were busy cleaning their catch. My children were fascinated as a man cut the head off of a beautiful yellowfin tuna and gutted it. I watched from afar, letting them both have a bit of independence on their vacation. After a few minutes though, my seven-year-old son screamed out, "Eww! I can see the mercury!" The fisherman looked at my child and then at me with horror and said, "There's no mercury in this fish!" Afterward, he muttered some words about how the world was being ruined by environmentalists and the like. I corrected my son and told him that he was not "seeing" the mercury, but that it was still in there. We are still laughing about that night, seven years later.

How much fish is safe to eat?

Mercury bioaccumulates. Therefore, in general, the larger the fish, the greater the concentration of mercury and the more you eat of them, the more that will accumulate in your body. Small fish haven't had enough time to accumulate as much of the toxin. Keep in mind that no amount of mercury is good for you. Mercury is a neurotoxin and can cause all kinds of problems in adults, including nervousness, muscle twitching, tremors, decreased cognition, and muscle atrophy. Mercury can affect a child's development and can cause fetal anomalies in pregnant women.[38] For this reason, children and pregnant women should be especially careful not to eat too much fish. The EPA set up guidelines based on body weight, designating the maximum mercury intake per day to be 0.1 micrograms per kilogram (2.2 pounds) per day. That equates to 7 micrograms per day, or 49 micrograms a week for a 70-kilogram (154-pound) person.

Fish that contain the highest levels of mercury include tilefish, shark, swordfish, king mackerel, and some types of tuna, including bigeye and ahi. Apologies to my fellow sushi lovers—these types of fish have been documented to contain over 100 micrograms of mercury in 4 ounces and should be avoided.

A middle tier of fish that contains between 40 and 80 micrograms of mercury per 4 ounces of cooked fish includes bluefin tuna and albacore tuna, canned white tuna (other than light tuna), yellowfin tuna, marlin, skipjack tuna, and lobster.

Lower levels of mercury have been found in salmon, light tuna (canned), pollock, tilapia, catfish, trout, and cod. Calamari (squid), clams, oysters, and shrimp also fall into this category. These species contain fewer than 40 micrograms of mercury per 4 ounces.

Research has been performed weighing the risk of mercury toxicity with the benefits of eating micronutrients and omega-3 fatty acids from fish[39], and the EPA-FDA recommendations for 2017 are for women and children to eat two to three servings of fish per week—one serving from the middle tier and the remaining serving(s) from the lowest tier.[40] Children under 10 should eat no more than three ounces of fish per week if the type of fish being eaten contains mercury. If you aren't sure how much this is, buy a small food scale. You'll be surprised at how little that actually is.

The Natural Resources Defense Council website (www.nrdc.org) lists types of fish and rates each variety by its level of typical mercury contamination. Familiarize yourself with this list and refer to it while you are shopping or eating out until you become more aware of which types of fish are safer to eat. Another great resource is www.SeafoodWatch.org. The easiest way to approach buying fish is to do some homework before going to the store. Pick out your favorite types of fish and figure out using a calculator what amount of fish you and your family can safely eat in a meal. Remember that the weights are based on the weight of the fish after it is cooked, so take that into consideration before your purchase.

The mercury levels listed are based on wild-caught fish. Farm-raised fish have a more controlled diet, and may therefore contain lower amounts of mercury than wild-caught fish. But these fish are typically raised in sectioned-off areas of offshore seawater, where they are potentially exposed to sources of pollution run-off from the land, including PCBs and dioxins.[41] This is important to consider since dioxins are very difficult to get rid of once they are in your body—their half-life in the human body has been measured to be 7.1 years![42] The most common varieties of fish now raised in farms include salmon, tilapia, sea bass, catfish, and cod. Farm-raised fish are fed feed, commonly including grains such as GMO corn and soy, which, as previously mentioned, may contain traces of pesticides and herbicides.[43] Farm-raised fish are also commonly fed antibiotics to keep diseases and pests under control.[44] With the exception of methyl mercury, most toxins are stored in the skin and fat, so it is best to trim off the fat and skin before eating any fish.[45]

The living conditions of farm-raised fish differ among countries and even between locations within a given country. It is not possible to generalize about the kinds of contaminants or the concentration level of contaminants in a given species of fish. I try to stay away from farm-raised fish, even though they are much lower in price.

Mussels have been shown to accumulate high levels of butyltin compounds, a chemical used in plastics and boat maintenance products. Unfortunately, this problem isn't going away anytime soon as these compounds don't degrade quickly and have been found in mussels even five years after bans on the chemicals have gone into effect in some countries.[46] Butyltin is an endocrine disruptor and a toxin that can impair the immune and central nervous systems. For this reason, it is best to limit your consumption of mussels.

Shrimp

Aside from fish, shrimp is the most commonly eaten seafood in the US. Would you believe that only 2% of the shrimp imported into this country is inspected by US regulatory agencies? Most shrimp is farm-raised and, like other types of fish, can be contaminated with a myriad of heavy metals and chemicals, including pesticides, dioxins and PCBs.[47] Shrimp contaminated with antibiotics banned in the US, such as chloramphenicol and nitrofuran, a known carcinogen,[48] arise on occasion.[49] Curiously, there are no research articles proving or disproving the safety of shrimp from the Gulf of Mexico after the notorious Gulf oil spill and subsequent spraying of over a million gallons of Corexit, a toxic oil dispersant. For this reason, I opt for fish from other locales. It's harder to find wild-caught shrimp in the grocery store, but it can always be ordered online.

Dairy counter

There are many different varieties of milk in the market. The most natural milk product is unprocessed "raw milk," only sold in select markets. Raw milk is better tasting and teeming with its own microbiome, which has beneficial health effects, including protecting children from the development of allergies.[50] But there is an increased risk of acquiring an infection from drinking raw milk.[51] Most retailers sell milk which has been pasteurized or ultra-pasteurized and homogenized.

Further processing creates subcategories of whole milk, including 2% milk, 1% milk, fat-free milk, lactose-free milk, and others.

Ultra-pasteurization has been around since 1993 in the US, but was used in Europe for many years before. During this process, milk is heated to 280°F with steam for two seconds and then rapidly cooled, killing virtually all of the bacteria within the milk. Most conventional milk and almost all organic milk in the US are now ultra-pasteurized. This technology increases the shelf life from one or two weeks to several months, which is efficient for a supermarket that doesn't want to worry about its milk spoiling too fast. During ultra-pasteurization, though, some milk proteins become denatured, meaning that they lose their structure, function, and perhaps digestibility. Perhaps even more important, nutritional value is diminished for milk that has been ultra-pasteurized.[52] Paying higher prices for organic milk that has been ultra-pasteurized may seem silly, yet these products do have fewer contaminants than their conventional alternatives.

Dairy cattle in the US are raised differently from beef cattle. Dairy cattle can be injected with a synthetic form of growth hormone called recombinant bovine somatotropin (rBGH), developed by Monsanto, which stimulates cattle, goats, and sheep to produce more milk. Milk produced by cows treated with rBGH is associated with increased levels of the hormone insulin-like growth factor (IGF-1). The American Cancer Society has questioned whether or not there is a link between IGF-1 and cancer.[53] To date, no direct link has been defined, but many countries, including the EU, have banned the use of rBGH. Due to a public backlash on this technology, there has been a drop-off of its use over the years.

Milk production in the US is also associated with markedly elevated levels of estrogen and progesterone, the female sex hormones. This may be related to the practice of artificially inseminating cattle while they are still producing milk from their previous pregnancies, which increases milk production. This practice occurs on conventional as well as organic farms. Many scientists have questioned whether or not the development of human cancers, such as breast, ovarian, and uterine cancer, is associated with the elevated female sex hormone levels in commercial milk.[54] Statistical analysis has also shown that men who drink whole milk increase their risk of developing and dying from prostate cancer.[55]

As a result of excessive milk production stimulated by rBGH administered from 60 to 305 days during the lactation period, cattle suffered a 25% increase in udder infections, known as mastitis, during this treatment period.[56] This painful condition can release pus and bacteria into the milk. If the milk is subsequently pasteurized, ultra-pasteurized, and homogenized, any potential pathogens in the milk are killed. However, the cattle raised in conventional farms are given antibiotics to treat mastitis. In addition, most dairy cattle are prophylactically injected with antibiotics each year to prevent them from getting the condition.[57] Residue of the circulating antibiotics in the cow's blood can then be secreted into the milk. As a result, some milk contains traces of antibiotics, some of which, the FDA recently discovered, have not even been approved for use in dairy cattle.[58]

Dairy products made from conventional milk, such as butter, cheese, sour cream, whipped cream, half-and-half, and heavy cream, are all made from the same dairy farms that inject their cattle with antibiotics, and yes, antibiotics have also been found in these foods. Organic milk producers are forbidden to treat mastitis with antibiotics, and therefore take greater care to ensure their animals are living in clean quarters and have healthy immune systems. Given the status of the US dairy market, I opt to feed my family organic dairy products, but sparingly.

Eggs and poultry

Many have seen horrifying images and videos of factory poultry farms where chickens live in such tight quarters that they have no room to move. Many factory hens never see natural daylight. With natural day-night cycles, egg-laying chickens and ducks lay more eggs during the summer season when daylight is longer. In the winter, they get a rest. With that in mind, factory poultry farmers artificially increase the daily light duration with lamps so their chickens will produce more eggs year-round. Instead of eating small plants and insects, factory chickens eat feed consisting of grains, including GMO corn.

Similar to cattle and fish, poultry farmers inject their birds with antibiotics to try and keep them free of disease.[59] Despite the use of antibiotics, chickens still get sick, probably because the pesticides and herbicides that lace their feed destroy the normal bacterial flora in the chickens' guts, leaving them with unhealthy intestinal biomes. Before the 1980s, people ate raw eggs without any fear of getting sick. Since then, though, the incidence of *Salmonella* infections has been on the rise. Today, signs in restaurants warn of eating eggs that aren't cooked thoroughly for fear of *Salmonella*. GMO feed with glyphosate residue has been implicated in disturbing the microbiomes of poultry, killing off beneficial bacteria and leaving behind those that are less susceptible to the chemical, such as *Salmonella* and *Clostridium*. This may in part explain the increased incidence of *Clostridium* and *Salmonella* infections in cattle, poultry farms, and conventional egg production factories.[60,61] However, the risk of salmonella persists in free-range and certified organic chicken populations.[62]

If you have the ability to raise your own chickens, I highly recommend it. Chickens are fun to watch, and collecting fresh eggs is a special gift each day. Otherwise, try to find a source of poultry and eggs that are not mass-produced from a factory farm. Be a savvy shopper and understand the deceptive labeling techniques used by some factory farms. Words like "all natural" mean nothing. Unfortunately, descriptions such as "free range," "cage free," and "naturally raised" are also misleading and don't really mean what they sound like they mean. It is best to ignore marketing ploys. A more useful label is one that specifies "organic eggs." In order to receive the organic label, the laying chickens aren't fed any GMO grain and are raised on land that has been free of pesticide and fertilizer use for at least three years. "Free-range" means the chickens have the ability to go outside, but this might mean that they are predominately housed indoors with access to just a small outdoor concrete slab. Making sure that your eggs are fully cooked will help eliminate the risk of acquiring a *Salmonella* infection.

Beans

Beans are nutritious, but can be dangerous if not prepared properly. Beans, particularly red kidney beans, need to be cooked at a high temperature by boiling for at least ten minutes before they are eaten. Bean plants, like other legumes, produce lectins, a class of compounds that has been shown to have antifungal, insecticidal, and antibacterial traits, among others.[63] Lectins can be toxic and inflammatory and can cause gastrointestinal symptoms such as nausea, vomiting, and diarrhea.[64] Before cooking beans in a slow cooker, you need to process them in one of two ways. Either precook the beans in a pressure cooker, or presoak the beans for twelve hours and then boil them for at least ten minutes. Either of these methods will neutralize the lectins and avoid toxicity. If neither of these options are possible, use canned beans instead of raw beans. Lima beans contain a compound called linamarin that will turn into the poisonous compound hydrogen cyanide after it is eaten.[65] Make sure to cook raw lima beans for at least ten minutes in boiling water to deactivate this toxin.

Grains

Milled wheat was the first processed food. Now, growing, harvesting, storing, and packaging wheat and flour is a highly complex process, with each step utilizing chemicals and, as mentioned earlier, irradiation. Wheat growers in the US and in many parts of the world apply Cycocel, a synthetic plant hormone that regulates growth characteristics of the wheat, to their fields.[66] Wheat plants, like many other grain crops, are killed immediately prior to harvest by spraying glyphosate on the field so that the grain can be harvested more easily. Glyphosate is subsequently absorbed by conventional wheat plants.[67] During wheat storage, malathion and pyrethrin are sprayed into the storage bins to protect the crop from moths and other insects. These chemicals have been implicated in toxic health effects, even in low concentrations.[68] Avoid these chemicals by eating organic grains.

Oats and oatmeal have many healthy effects on the body's cardiovascular system, such as lowering blood pressure and modestly lowering cholesterol levels.[69] Organic and conventional oats and oat-based breakfast cereals and snacks may contain elevated concentrations of the toxin ochratoxin A (OTA), produced by a mold known to grow on oats and other grains.[70] The research on this toxin is not yet complete, but it is suspected that this toxin can cause kidney cancer.[71] The International Agency for Research on Cancer (a branch of the World Health Organization) classifies this toxin as a possible human carcinogen.

Rice

Rice has been found to aggregate heavy metals. Depending on the soil the rice is grown in, these metals can include zinc, calcium, manganese, and iron, which are nutritious for our body. Unfortunately, toxic metals, including cadmium, mercury, tungsten, and arsenic, can also be absorbed by rice plants. As soils become more and more polluted by industrial waste, rice crops are becoming more and more contaminated with these toxic metals. This is a health concern for rice grown in the US as well as in countries such as China, where industrial heavy-metal contamination has led to elevated cadmium, lead, and mercury levels in the rice.[72]

Expand your knowledge

For the most part, the US food industry has done an excellent job keeping the general public safe from pathogens that can potentially infect whole foods. But as understanding of the microbiome increases, be aware of what you are eating and how it will affect the beneficial bacteria that live in your gut. Try to make the best choices you can given the information that you have, and keep yourself updated and educated on the current status of the food supply. Learning about the food you eat is an ongoing but worthwhile process.

PART II
CONVENIENCES

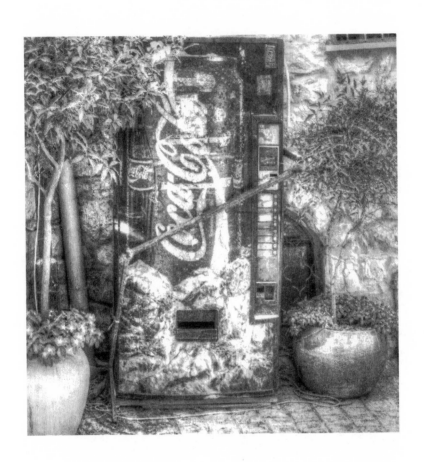

Chapter 4
PROCESSED FOODS

If it were possible to only eat ripe, fresh, whole foods, we would all be better off. But most everything sold in a supermarket has been processed to some extent. As discussed in the previous chapter, farm produce usually needs to be processed to last from harvest through storage, shipping, and display. Even people who grow their own produce need to process food for storage.

Canned foods

Canned fruits and vegetables are not as nutritious as their freshly picked counterparts, as processing destroys some of their vitamins and other nutrients. But the nutritional loss from processing doesn't make these products harmful. The quality of the fruit or vegetable chosen for processing and the materials chosen for packaging are both very important.

Cans, one of the oldest methods for storing food, can be made of steel, tin-coated steel, or aluminum. There has been an interesting evolution of aluminum cans. Initially, cans were implicated in lead poisoning, as the sealing process utilized a lead-containing metallic alloy. Health issues also arose from the corrosion of the tin lining by acidic foods, which caused toxicity. As a solution, cans were lined with a plastic coating containing BPA. Now a known endocrine disruptor, BPA can leach into the food contained within the can.[1] Acidic foods and those cans exposed to increased temperatures will result in more BPA leaching out into the food.[2] Just as with plastic bottles, chemical companies have made new BPA-free can liners. But many of these new chemicals are also turning out to be endocrine disruptors.[3] It is preferable to purchase canned vegetables and fruits in glass jars, especially acidic foods, such as tomato sauce. If a can's lid is not vacuum-sealed, toss it out. Botulism caused by *Clostridium* bacteria can contaminate improperly canned food and result in severe illness.

Frozen foods are processed, but less so than canned goods. There is no concern for plastic-related toxins dissolving into frozen food, and frozen vegetables contain much less salt than their canned varieties. Avoid consuming traces of pesticides and herbicides by eating frozen organic fruits and vegetables rather than conventionally grown produce, as with canned goods.

Sweeteners

There are so many sweeteners on the market it's dizzying. Along with aroma, sweetness is the first sense we appreciate from food we eat. Unfortunately, too much sugar is bad for your health and can lead to inflammatory disease, as well as obesity and diabetes. With recommended dietary restrictions on sugar intake, the artificial sweetener industry has developed on the premise that synthetic sugars are a healthier alternative to the real thing.

Refined white sugar, brown sugar, and raw sugar are processed materials derived from the sugar cane plant. Refined white sugars are repeatedly boiled to remove all of the molasses, whereas the raw sugar varieties retain a small amount of residual molasses. Raw sugar has a little more flavor and a coarser texture than refined sugar, with no significant difference in the nutritional value. Now, however, refined sugar is commonly produced by processing sugar beets, a GMO-approved plant. If you prefer refined white sugar, buy a product that is labeled "pure cane sugar" to avoid the GMO variety and any toxic residues they may contain.

If you want to limit your sugar intake, sweeten your food with other natural sweeteners. Honey is sweet, nutritious, and has antibacterial and antiviral properties.[4] Other "natural" sweeteners, including agave, maple syrup, and stevia are all processed foods. Agave nectar is marketed as a natural, low-glycemic sweetener, originating from the blue agave plant.

However, "raw" agave is a highly processed syrup with the highest concentration of fructose of any of the sweeteners, including high-fructose corn syrup.

A species of leafy green plant called Stevia, native to parts of the American Southwest and South America, contains a naturally sweet compound. Although the stevia plant leaves themselves are not approved by the FDA, a chemical isolated from the plant, called rebaudioside A (Rab A), or stevioside, has been approved as a dietary supplement in the US and is used to create powders such as stevia and Truvia, both zero-calorie sweeteners. Some studies have shown stevioside to have a very low toxicity[5] when used in moderation. However, a few early studies suggested that the stevioside extract can do damage to the male reproductive system, affecting fertility. In addition, a metabolite of stevioside produced in the intestine, known as steviol, has the potential to be genotoxic.[6] Unlike the US, the EU does not permit the use of Stevia.[7]

Artificial sweeteners began with the invention of saccharine in the late 1800s. Since then, the FDA has approved five artificial sweeteners, including saccharin, acesulfame, aspartame, neotame, and sucralose. These chemicals, sold individually in little colorful packets (pink, blue, green, yellow, etc.), can also be found in all kinds of foods labeled zero-calorie, one-calorie, low-calorie, and diet. Synthetic sugars are sweeter than sugar and are addicting. Because the sensation of sweetness is not associated with any intake of energy, the brain doesn't recognize that the body has taken in nutrition and so it continues to crave food.[8] This is perhaps the reason why artificial sweeteners are associated with weight gain instead of weight loss.[9] Although the National Cancer Institute has stated that there is no clear association between artificial sweeteners and cancer in humans, research studies have shown associations between artificial sweeteners and cancer in animals.[10] A link between cancer development in humans or any other adverse health effects from any of the approved artificial sweeteners in the US has not been proven.[11]

If artificial sweeteners don't help you lose weight and there is even a small potential for a negative health effect, why use them? What I've typically heard from users is that sugar isn't sweet enough. The good news is that if you have been addicted to these sweeteners and you cut them out of your diet, over time, you will eventually regain a normal sense for sweetness. But be aware that because of increasing public scrutiny, food companies are now using obscure names to hide these chemicals in ingredient lists.

Much of the information written about high-fructose corn syrup (HFCS) is propaganda put out by the Corn Refiners Association, a very politically active and wealthy group which has created an incredible market for itself. It's absolutely amazing to think about how this one sweetener has dominated the processed food industry. Gone are the days when cola was made with cane sugar, except in other countries.

High-fructose corn syrup isn't a natural sugar, but rather a chemical extracted from the corn plant. Biochemically, refined sugar is typically 50% glucose and 50% fructose, but HFCS has a much higher percentage of fructose, hence the name "high fructose."[12]

HFCS is sweeter and cheaper to produce than cane sugar. Fructose is sweet, but isn't metabolized by the body as easily as glucose. When fructose enters the bloodstream and passes into the liver, it triggers the production of fat.[13] Too much dietary fructose therefore can lead to metabolic disturbance, and has been implicated as causing chronic health conditions, including obesity, diabetes, heart disease, and cancer of the pancreas, liver, and colon.[14] Some researchers speculate that the ingestion of HFCS may cause energy depletion in the intestinal cells that absorb them, leading to inflammation and other immune reactions, contributing to leaky gut syndrome.[15] HFCS may now be derived from GMO corn, introducing a whole new level of potential contamination, including pesticide and herbicide residue. As if that weren't enough, the toxic heavy metal mercury has also been documented as a contaminant in the production of HFCS.[16] Read packaging labels and try to limit the ingestion of foods containing HFCS as much as possible.

Synthetic fats

Synthetic fats may be as bad (if not worse) for your health as synthetic sugars. Unfortunately, identifying these chemical additives on ingredient panels can be challenging. Synthetic fat production began with the creation of Crisco, the first shortening to be entirely made from vegetable oil. Crisco, that old-time kitchen staple with which Grandma used to make amazing pie crust, was introduced to the market in the mid-1920s, and by the thirties and forties, everyone who was anyone used Crisco. Free cookbooks were even handed out with Crisco recipes. Crisco became the ingredient of higher society! What an amazing marketing feat to have been able to convince people living on farms that they needed to buy a synthetic fat for cooking instead of using the butter and lard they could render from their own animals. Some think that the cardiovascular health problems in the US began with the introduction of processed vegetable oils and fats into our diet.[17]

Since Crisco, many synthetic fats have hit the market. The best-known synthetic fat in production today is known as olestra (OleanTM), which was approved for use in foods by the FDA in 1996. This product was created by the NutraSweet Company by chemically binding a sugar molecule (sucrose) to a fatty acid, resulting in a sucrose-polyester compound that looks, tastes, and feels like fat. Our bodies do not have the necessary enzymes to break down this material and it passes through the digestive tract without being digested or absorbed.[18] In larger amounts, this synthetic material can function as a stool softener and cause malabsorption symptoms, such as abdominal cramping, excessive gas, and loose bowel movements. Olestra intake has also been associated with decreased intestinal absorption of some nutrients and vitamins.[19]

Simplesse, a synthetic "fat" made from egg and dairy whey protein, is currently used in commercially prepared salad dressings, sauces, yogurts, and other cold foods—it can't be used in hot foods. Simplesse was created by breaking down whey protein molecules into tiny microparticles, one micron in diameter. The tiny size of the particles gives the product its fatty texture and other properties. At the present time, research for potential health effects on this material is lacking. These microparticles are highly processed and I prefer eating packaged foods without nebulous ingredients such as whey protein concentrate, milk protein, or dairy protein, all approved labels for "Simplesse."

Trans fats, which are fatty acids created by the hydrogenation of unsaturated oils, are inexpensive, stable, synthetic vegetable oils that increase the shelf life of the products that contain them. Trans fats have a less greasy feel than other fats and have been used in all kinds of processed foods for many years. Research has shown trans fats to be associated with the development of cancer, diabetes, heart disease, obesity, and many other inflammatory diseases.[20,21] Because trans fats have been associated with coronary heart disease and sudden cardiac death,[18] the FDA began requiring labeling of all foods containing trans fats in 2006. Under public pressure, the FDA in 2013 made a preliminary determination that partially hydrogenated oils (trans fats) are no longer generally recognized as safe (GRAS) in human food. A governmental ban on trans fats, approved in 2015, will require US food manufacturers to remove trans fats from all food products by 2018. In preparation, many processed food companies have already changed their recipes and replaced trans fats with other materials thought to be less hazardous.

One such material that food companies are now using is known as interesterified fat. These synthetic fats are generated by using naturally occurring fat molecules, referred to as triacylglycerols, which are composed of three fatty acids attached to a glycerol molecule. Our digestive enzymes recognize these components and are able to break them down during the digestive process. The length and composition of the fatty acids give a fat molecule its physical properties and biochemical characteristics. Using this knowledge, interesterified fats are created biochemically by swapping or rearranging the location and length of the fatty acid chains to create unique molecules with desirable properties, such as a long shelf life. But as research accumulates, these products are being discovered to cause significant health problems.[22] There are currently no labeling requirements for interesterified fats. If an ingredient says 0 grams trans fat or no trans fat, check the ingredients and see if the product contains vegetable oil. If it does, you can be certain that the product contains either fully hydrogenated vegetable oil, interesterified fats, or less than 0.5g per serving of partially hydrogenated vegetable oil, which is considered a small enough amount to be labeled 0 grams.

Many vegetable oils are highly processed foods extracted from seeds and other plant materials, margarine included. Margarine was first created in the early 1800s as an inexpensive substitute for butter. Early margarines were made from animal fat, but now, margarine is manufactured from a vegetable oil substrate. The manufacturing process is not as secret as the process for creating high-fructose corn syrup and can be found on the Internet. It is as follows:

Recipe to create Margarine

1. Seeds from plants such as corn, cotton, soybean, and safflower are collected and the oils are extracted by utilizing hexane, an organic solvent. (Organic in this context means that it contains carbon atoms— six carbon atoms in the case of hexane). The process of extraction results in free radicals.
2. The oil is steamed to remove most of the impurities, thereby destroying the vitamins and natural antioxidants found in the oil.
3. Hydrogen gas is bubbled through the liquid oil in the presence of a catalyst (usually nickel). This forces unsaturated fatty acids to become saturated and solid. The more complete the hydrogenation process, the firmer the finished product. Margarine undergoes partial hydrogenation to make it semi-solid. The resulting lump of gray grease contains a high content of trans fats.
4. Emulsifiers are mixed in with the mixture to remove lumps and the mixture is bleached to change the gray color to white.
5. A second steam cleaning removes any odors that may be attributed to residual chemicals in the mixture.
6. Chemists add artificial colors and yellow dye to make the product appear more palatable. The final product is then packaged and marketed as a healthier alternative to butter!

In my home, we use natural fats. Organic butter, coconut oil, olive oil, and even lard are my preferred cooking fats. All lard, however, is not equal. A healthy, pasture-raised, organically raised pig that hasn't been raised on GMO grain, antibiotics, or hormones is a preferable source of lard. As animal fat accumulates toxins, eating or cooking with lard will potentially expose one to the toxins an animal was exposed to during its life. If you are going to cook with lard, make it yourself by rendering the pork fat and then storing it in a jar. Lard can be frozen, refrigerated, or placed in a clean canning jar on the shelf. If the fat is properly rendered, lard should last for up to a year in the refrigerator or three years in a freezer.

Nitrates/nitrites

Nitrates in and of themselves are not harmful, but what our body does with nitrates may or may not be dangerous to health. In the mouth, bacteria and other enzymes turn nitrates into nitrites. In turn, nitrites may form one of two different chemical compounds in the body: nitric oxide or nitrosamine. Nitric oxide is a chemical the body uses in specific concentrations and in specific tissues to derive benefit, notably by relaxing arteries, reducing blood pressure and improving circulation.[23] Conversely, nitrosamines are associated with cancer, particularly along the gastrointestinal tract, including the esophagus, stomach, colon, and rectum.[24,25]

So what decides the fate of the nitrites and whether they will be converted to nitric oxide or nitrosamines? Nitrates are found in many types of vegetables, such as celery. When ingested in vegetables, nitrates may be converted into nitric oxide, which can significantly improve cardiovascular health.[26] Nitrites, however, form nitrosamines when they are subjected to high heat or when they enter an acidic environment in the presence of proteins.[27] Nitrates and nitrites are commonly used to preserve processed meats such as hot dogs and bacon so the heat from a skillet, grill, or broiler can be the perfect laboratory for the production of nitrosamines. In addition, the acidic environment of the stomach can produce nitrosamines from cold processed meat.

Check labels to see if your package of smoked meat says, "No nitrates added." Look for a disclaimer such as, "Except those occurring naturally in celery juice," or something similar. Alternatively, there may be celery powder, celery juice, or celery salt listed in the ingredients panel. This is a deceptive tactic that the food companies use to hide nitrates. Even though celery juice is a source of nitrates, a product can contain celery juice and sport a "No nitrates added" label. The nitrate source is irrelevant. Nitrates + protein + high heat = nitrosamines.

The government has recognized the potential carcinogenic nature of nitrates and has issued two requirements on food suppliers. For one, food manufacturers are now required to limit the amount of nitrites and nitrates they use in processed meats. In addition, food manufacturers are required to add vitamin C to their products, which has been shown to inhibit nitrosamine formation.[28] It would stand to reason, therefore, that if you ingest vitamin C with your bacon at breakfast, perhaps by taking a supplement or by drinking a glass of juice containing vitamin C, this will also help inhibit the production of nitrosamines. In general, processed meat eaten today contains much less nitrates and nitrites than it did a few decades ago. But even so, the World Health Organization recently declared processed meat as carcinogenic to humans due to nitrosamine formation as well as the formation of other toxic compounds during processing and digestion.[29]

The ingredient panel

Aside from the synthetic sugars, synthetic fats, and nitrates placed into food to make it last longer, taste better, or in other ways "design" it, thousands of additional other chemicals have been approved for processed foods. The list expands yearly.

In order to limit your exposure to these chemicals, read the ingredient panel on each packaged, processed food. Most added chemicals will be listed in the ingredients, but some will not. Even if you have purchased the same food by the same company for years, periodically check the ingredient panel for changes, especially if the packaging has changed. Companies frequently change ingredients and add or subtract chemicals to improve the flavor, appearance, texture, or shelf life of a product. Packaging may add words such as "New bolder flavor," "More creamy," "Now fewer calories," "Now extra thick and tasty," etc. If the package wording or design has changed, recheck the ingredients to make sure you are still comfortable eating the product.

The ingredient panel includes two important components. One is the nutritional section and the other is the actual list of ingredients. Both sections include very important information, and the more you get comfortable reading and interpreting these panels, the better able you will be to critically evaluate what you are eating. This really is an important process when you are a consumer of processed foods. The nutritional panel has very limited, basic information on the nutritional value of the food, including calories, fat, carbohydrates, and protein content. It also lists the amount of sodium. The more nebulous portion of the nutritional panel is the list of ingredients.

A popular prepared food has an ingredient panel that lists the following:

> **Ingredients:** Enriched macaroni product (wheat flour, niacin, ferrous sulfate (iron), thiamin mononitrate (vitamin B1); riboflavin (vitamin B2), folic acid); Cheese sauce mix: whey, cheddar cheese, whey protein concentrate, maltodextrin, salt, modified food starch (contains less than 2% of sodium tripolyphosphate, citric acid, cream, skim milk, spice, sodium diacetate, cellulose gel, cellulose gum, cayenne pepper, vinegar, salt, garlic, sodium phosphate, sodium acetate, paprika, yeast extract, natural flavor, dried garlic, disodium insinuate and disodium guanylate, paprika extract, beta carotene (color)).

If one removes "food" from this recipe, including wheat flour, whey, cheddar cheese, cream, skim milk, cayenne pepper, vinegar, salt, and garlic, the remaining ingredients include:

> Niacin, ferrous sulfate (Iron), thiamin mononitrate (vitamin B1); riboflavin (vitamin B2), folic acid, maltodextrin, modified food starch, sodium tripolyphosphate, citric acid, sodium diacetate, cellulose gel, cellulose gum, sodium phosphate, sodium acetate, natural flavor, disodium insinuate and disodium guanylate, beta carotene (color).

The vitamins listed on an ingredient panel are synthetic nutritional supplements added to processed food to seemingly create a more nutritious product (Table 4). Although these chemical supplements are designed to mimic natural vitamins, the body's ability to absorb a synthetic vitamin and the vitamin concentration within a processed food can differ substantially from its ability to absorb vitamins within a naturally occurring food source, such as a vegetable.

After removing synthetic vitamins and minerals from the list in the example, the remaining ingredients include:

Maltodextrin, modified food starch, sodium tripolyphosphate, citric acid, sodium diacetate, cellulose gel, cellulose gum, sodium phosphate, sodium acetate, natural flavor, disodium insinuate and disodium guanylate.

Many of these remaining ingredients have no nutritional value and are simply not food.

Table 4. List of synthetic vitamins

Reinoic acid, retinol, retinal - Vitamin A
Beta carotene - (Converted to Vitamin A)
Thiamin mononitrate - Vitamin B1
Riboflavin - Vitamin B2
Niacin, niacinamide - Vitamin B3
Pantothenic acid - Vitamin B5
Pyridoxine, pyridoxamine, pyridoxal - Vitamin B6
Biotin - Vitamin B7
Cyanocobalamin, hydroxycobalamin, methylcobalamin - Vitamin
      B12
Ascorbic acid - Vitamin C
Calciferol in the forms of cholecalciferol, ergocalciferol - Vitamin
      D3, Vitamin D2
Alpha tocopherol - Vitamin E
Folic acid - Vitamin B9
Phylloquinone, menaquinone - Vitamin K

Compare the nutritional panel of the prior processed food to an organic alternative:

Ingredients: *Organic wheat macaroni, cheddar cheese (cultured pasteurized milk, salt, non-animal* *enzymes), whey, nonfat milk, butter, salt, cultured whole milk, sodium phosphate, annatto extract for color.*

After removing foods, the ingredients remaining include:

non-animal enzymes and sodium phosphate

Non-animal enzymes include a distillate of vegetable-based enzymes, requiring a chemical process for purification. Sodium phosphate is a generic term for salts created by mixing the elements sodium and phosphorus. Sodium phosphates are common chemicals used in food processing to emulsify mixtures so that cheeses and oils blend, improving food texture. Other common emulsifiers include polysorbate 80 and carboxymethylcellulose.

Have you ever given a thought to what your body does with the chemicals added to processed food? Even emulsifiers approved for organic food have been implicated in disturbing the intestinal microbiome and may also contribute to intestinal inflammation and metabolic syndromes.[30] It would be safe to say that no one is completely sure of the health effects of the thousands of approved chemical agents or how they interact when mixed together. Even though these chemicals may have been approved by the FDA, approach them with caution and limit how much you ingest. It may not be possible to completely eradicate these chemicals from your diet, but as you become more conscious of what you are eating, you will naturally gravitate toward whole food instead of food with additives and chemical substitutes.

The USDA and FDA require the labeling of most ingredients in processed foods so that consumers can sort of know what they are eating. Unfortunately, though, there are exceptions. Many ingredients do not require labeling, particularly if they are placed into a food product in very small quantities. For example, if a food contains 0.5 grams of trans fat per serving, the food label can deceptively read "0" grams of trans fat! My suggestion would be to limit ingestion of processed foods as much as you can. If you do choose to buy pre-packaged foods, opt for products labeled with an expiration date that would be expected if you made a similar product at home. For example, if you baked a batch of cookies, how many days would you expect them to keep fresh? It is only through the addition of preservatives and the use of synthetic fats that a package of cookies in the market can stay fresh for six months or longer.

GMOs

In 2016, a labeling law was signed by President Obama requiring manufacturers to disclose which of their processed foods contain GMO ingredients. However, the label can be hard to decipher. In fact, the label can be in QR code, decodable only with an app on a smart phone. Alternatively, manufacturers can provide a 1-800 number for consumers to call to find out if a product contains GMO ingredients. Unfortunately, this labeling law is not nearly as helpful to the public as one that would require an easily recognizable packaging symbol.

So now, for example, if you are eating a food that contains GMO corn as an ingredient, it will be listed simply as "corn." Similarly, labels will not specify if high-fructose corn syrup is created from GMO corn. The USDA offers a voluntary government labeling and certification program for food that does not contain genetically modified ingredients. Companies that choose to apply GMO-free labeling to their food products can receive a USDA process-verified label, proving the product is GMO-free.

As of now, the only approved GMO foods are corn, soybean, sugar beets, Hawaiian papaya, and cotton. The ingredients created from these foods, however, are extensive, and are listed in Table 5.

Table 5. Products created from GMO ingredients

Corn derivatives:

High-frustose corn syrup	Corn syrup
Baking powder	Caramel color
Citric acid	Corn meal
Corn starch	Dextrin

Maltodextrin	Monosodium glutamate (MSG)
Sorbitol	Polysorbate 80 and others
Sodium erythorbate	Sorbitan
Sorbitan monostearate	Starch
Sucrfalose	Sweet'N Low
Vanilla extract	Vinegar, distilled white
Xanthan gum	Xylitol

Vitamins used for enrichment in foods, including Vitamin C

Soybeans:

Soy flour
Lecithin
Soy sauce
Soy protein isolates and concentrations

Sugar beets:

Sugar in different forms, including granulated sugar, icing sugar, rock sugar, and gelling sugar. (Any processed food that lists "sugar" instead of "cane sugar" is most likely from GMO sugar beets, including cookies, cakes, ice cream, donuts, baking mixes, candy, juice, and yogurt.)
Inverted sugar syrup
Caramel color
Citric acid
Nutritional yeast

Nanoparticles

Nanoparticles are the product of a technology that is being used not only for the food industry, but also for many other industries, including personal care products, medicine, electronics, clothing, sports equipment, fertilizers, and pesticides. Within the food industry, nanotechnology is being used in the preparation of processed foods, in food packaging, and in food storage.

Nanoparticles are tiny particles measuring one-billionth of a meter, or 1/1000th the size of a microparticle. Nanotechnology takes advantage of physical property changes that various compounds and elements exhibit while in this tiny form. For example, copper and zinc, both opaque, shiny metals, become transparent when they are turned into nanoparticles. Titanium dioxide is a common nanoparticle used in the food industry. When nanoparticles are mixed into a food item, the industry refers to the resulting product as a "nanofood."

Proponents of this technology say that in foods, nanoparticles can have beneficial effects, such as boosting the bioavailability of nutrients, extending food shelf life, and improving taste. Nanoparticles can also be used to deter and detect bacterial contamination.

This is not a new technology. In fact, if you enjoy Heinz ketchup, you have been ingesting nanoparticles for years. Some are old enough to remember watching the Heinz ketchup commercial showing the slow descent of ketchup from a ketchup bottle onto a hamburger while the Carly Simon song "Anticipation" played. Now, ketchup comes out of the bottle easily because of the introduction of nanoparticles to the recipe.

Here is a list of some companies that have been integrating nanotechnology into their food products:

Heinz	Nestlé
The Hershey Co.	Unilever
Campina	General Mills
Friesland Foods	Kraft
Cargill	PepsiCo
ConAgra Foods	

Not all companies have had success with their new products. For example, Dunkin' Donuts was criticized for using titanium dioxide on their powdered donuts, and stopped using it. (The FDA allows up to 1% titanium dioxide nanoparticles to be placed into a food without any labeling requirement.)

Each individual company is solely responsible for the decision to use nanotechnology in food preparation or packaging and there are no requirements for divulging its use. Even organic foods are permitted to contain nanoparticles. Some of the more common compounds used in packaged food recipes include titanium oxide, titanium dioxide, silicon oxide, and zinc oxide. These nanoparticles, when mixed into recipes, make the products look better and increase shelf life. Ice cream becomes smoother and richer. Whipped cream becomes extra creamy. Salad dressings and sauces gain a more intense flavor.

Due to their tiny size, nanoparticles can pass directly from the body's intestine into the bloodstream. From there, they can pass freely to all of the cells in the body, even the brain and the testes.[31,32] Research has shown that it may take four months for the body to clear silver nanoparticles following exposure. Exceptions to this are the brain and testes, which, disturbingly, showed no clearance of nanoparticles, even after four months.[33] If it takes four months to clear silver nanoparticles from the body after exposure, imagine the bioaccumulation that would occur with repeated exposure. Outside the food industry, there are many different chemicals that are now being turned into nanoparticles, and many of them have been proven to be biopersistent.

Nanoparticles may harm some of our body's cells. Although not much published research has been done on living cells, one experiment exposed rats to repeated doses of nanoparticles through food. Researchers found that the testes of these rats were abnormal, indicating that there was a significant negative impact on the production of sperm from nanoparticles.[34] Could nanoparticles be one of the reasons why fertility rates among men has been decreasing in the US? More research needs to be done to better assess the physiologic effects of nanoparticles on human male fertility and other organ systems.

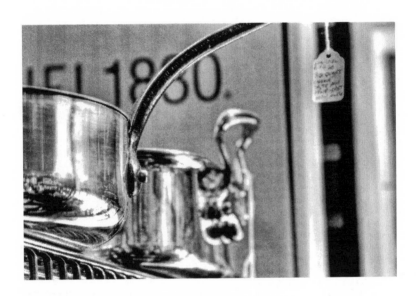

Chapter 5

FOOD PREPARATION AND PACKAGING

Almost all materials that come into contact with food can react with it. These reactions may be minimal or significant, depending on the type of food, the composition of the wrapping or cooking material, and the prevailing atmosphere or environment—particularly temperature.[1] Cooking food is akin to alchemy. You should consider your pot or pan a laboratory where chemical reactions occur as a result of mixing ingredients together with applied heat.

Kitchen products

Many different elements and compounds have been used to create tools to assist with food preparation. Included among these products are bowls for mixing and utensils for beating, stirring, cutting, and spreading. Pots, pans, Pyrex, and casserole dishes are available for cooking and baking. If you prepare food at home, take a stroll around your kitchen and open up a few cupboards. I'm sure you will see a wide selection of shapes and sizes of all of the above.

What makes one kitchen product more desirable for use than another? Perhaps you enjoy your plastic mixing bowls because they're light and colorful. You can easily recognize what you have placed in each bowl because of the color of the bowl. Or maybe you prefer a set of glass bowls because you like the visibility of the ingredients and the clean look of glass. Why do you like your favorite pot or pan? Is it light? Does it have a nonstick surface? Does it heat your food evenly? These are all typical attributes that a cook may seek out when shopping for cookware. When considering your health, though, the list might change a bit. Instead of convenience and appearance, more attention to the materials themselves will help limit the number and concentration of contaminants that can leach out into food.

Pots and pans with nonstick surfaces

Perhaps one of the most controversial items in the kitchen is the nonstick surface found on cookware. It makes cleanup a breeze, allows one to easily manipulate the ingredients being cooked, and prevents tearing or otherwise compromising the appearance of the finished product. Do you know what goes into making a nonstick surface?

The nonstick concept originated with the discovery of a fluoropolymer called Teflon. Teflon is the brand name for a slippery chemical called polytetrafluoroethylene (PTFE), which was created and first marketed in 1945 by the DuPont Company. This chemical was subsequently applied to cookware in 1956 by a French engineer, who in that same year founded the Tefal Corporation (T-fal) with his wife. Since then, many companies have developed other fluoropolymers that are different from PTFE.

Fluoropolymers have been used in the production of cookware for a long time now, and over that time span, have been implicated in some disturbing health effects. One of the most publicized of these concerns was the recognition of the biopersistence of a contaminant in PTFE, a chemical used in its production known as perfluorooctanoid acid (PFOA). Since the 1990s, this compound (also called "C8") has been found at low levels throughout the environment and in the U.S. population as measured in the blood supply.[2] It will remain in people for a very long time, for there is no way for the human body to eliminate it. PFOA has been associated with many adverse health effects in people and animals.

People with occupational exposure to higher levels of PFOA have been shown to have an increased incidence of ulcerative colitis and rheumatoid arthritis.[3] Research has been conducted to study the health effects of PFOA at lower concentrations, but these studies are much fewer in number. Links have been made between PFOA exposure and kidney cancer and bladder cancer,[4] non-hepatitis liver disease,[5] and thyroid disease.[6] Certainly concentration, chronicity, and individual immunologic response would more than likely factor into any one person's potential for developing disease when exposed to a chemical such as PFOA.

In addition to being used in cookware, PFOA has been used in all types of waterproof, breathable fabrics and membranes. Despite the hundreds of recreational and industrial uses of PFOA, DuPont no longer produces it because of its biopersistence and toxicity.

A second chemical compound with properties similar to PFOA used in the production of fluoropolymers is perfluorooctyl sulfonate (PFOS). This compound was also found to be widespread in blood samples throughout the general U.S. population.[7] In the 1990s, this raised concerns about both its biopersistence and its toxicity. As a result, 3M, the primary manufacturer of PFOS, stopped producing this chemical.

Many of these types of chemicals have been phased out since 2006, but some companies continue to produce them and use them in their products. Take a moment to think about this. These toxic, biopersistent chemicals were leaching into our foods for just about fifty years before we discovered they were harmful to our health and phased them out! To me, that's mind-boggling. So, if you look around your kitchen and see that you have old Teflon pans, what should you do with them? My suggestion would be to toss them out and buy something else, particularly if the surface of your pan is scratched or worn in any way.

Are you aware that if you overheat a nonstick pan, you'll release chemicals from its coating into the air?[8] Back in the 1970s it was discovered that pet birds could die if they breathed in these toxic chemicals.[9,10] In people, inhaling these gases can cause a chemical pneumonitis (pneumonia) with flu-like symptoms.[11] This is a potential short-term toxic effect from using a nonstick pan. The long-term toxic effects are very difficult to isolate, given that we are exposed to so many different toxins and contaminants in our environment on a regular basis. As there are plenty of alternative materials to cook with, I avoid using this type of cookware.

Aluminum

Aluminum is the third most prevalent element on Earth, but its ingestion and/or absorption has been implicated in the development of Alzheimer's disease and osteoporosis. Although the research has been muddied over the past forty years with conflicting scientific results, a recent meta-analysis of the data compiled from various studies—including more than 10,000 patients with long-term exposure to aluminum— found that individuals chronically exposed to aluminum were 71% more likely to develop Alzheimer's disease.[12] Aluminum is a known neurotoxin,[13] and aluminum deposits have been found in the brains of patients with Alzheimer's disease.[14] Aluminum has also been shown to be a metalloestrogen and can cause hormonal effects. Breast cancer has been associated with aluminum exposure through the use of antiperspirants.[15] In June 2011, the Joint Food and Agriculture Organization, a joint committee of the United Nations and the World Health Organization (WHO), proposed a dietary intake limit of two mg/kg of aluminum from all sources, including drinking water and food. Calculating one's ingestion of aluminum daily is unrealistic, and unfortunately many populations in the world have exposures that are higher than this limit.[16,17] The greatest exposure to aluminum may come from food, depending on one's diet.[16,18] In one study from China, even leafy green vegetables were shown to have high levels of aluminum, absorbed from the soil.[19]

Your choice of cookware may also contribute to the quantity of aluminum you ingest. There has been concern over the years that aluminum can leach into your food from a pot or pan in two ways: mechanically and chemically. By using a sharp or hard utensil such as a metal fork or a spatula on an aluminum pan, you can scrape off and dislodge particles of aluminum by abrasion. If the pan is worn or contains pits and scratches, scraping the pan will release even more aluminum particles. Aluminum can also leach into food through chemical interaction, particularly with acidic and salty foods.[20]

There are two types of aluminum pots and pans on the market: anodized and non-anodized. Anodized cookware has a thin layer of aluminum oxide on its surface. This layer makes the surface more durable and less likely to flake off and corrode. Therefore, if you prefer to cook with aluminum pans, anodized aluminum cookware is a safer product. Anodized cookware conducts heat quickly and its surface is nonstick and scratch-resistant. Calphalon is a well-known, respected brand of anodized nonstick aluminum cookware.

Copper

During a trip to Brazil a number of years ago, my wife and I stopped by the side of a windy mountain road where an artisan had set up a stand to sell beautiful handcrafted copper products. We purchased a set of beautiful copper pots and pans from him. The oversized pans were seemingly perfect for cooking and serving large groups of people. My wife and I both loved the rustic look of the cookware.

Unfortunately, what I have since learned is that the use of copper pots and pans for cooking is dangerous to your health. Just as aluminum can leach into food, the same is true of copper pots and pans.[21] Large amounts of copper, either in a single dose or over a short period of time, can leach into your food and be poisonous. It has been suggested that Alzheimer's disease may be caused by excessive copper ingestion.[22]

The amount of copper required to create toxicity, however, is unclear. It is true that a small amount of copper as a trace mineral is important for one's everyday health, but cooking with a copper pot is not recommended. For this reason, most commercially sold copper cookware is surface-coated with a safer metal so that the copper doesn't come into contact with one's food. These pots and pans are safe to use as long as the coating remains intact. Our copper pots and pans are now only used for decoration.

Stainless steel and cast iron

Most cookware today is made of either stainless steel or cast iron. The most common metals that can leach into food from these materials are iron, nickel, and chromium.[23] Large amounts of any of them can be toxic. Cooking acidic foods, such as tomato sauce, have been shown to leach nickel and chromium, which can cause health concerns in some populations. Nickel, in particular, can cause allergic contact dermatitis, a skin condition that is increasing in incidence.[24] If you or someone in your family has a known nickel allergy or suffers skin rashes due to allergic contact dermatitis, you should not prepare a meal with nickel-plated stainless steel cookware.

Ceramic, enamel, and glass

Ceramic and enameled cookware are excellent to cook with and are considered safe as long as there are no painted surfaces inside the cooking vessel. Some paint pigments may contain traces of lead or cadmium, which can also leach into food.[25,26] Heavy metal toxicity is a more significant concern with pottery and cookware purchased in other countries, because in the United States and Canada regulations exist to restrict the amount of lead and cadmium that may be used in the manufacture of cookware. These regulations do not necessarily exist in other countries, so be careful when importing cooking materials.

Products made of other materials

Titanium products entered the market several years ago and are exorbitantly priced. These products vary from pure titanium cookware to titanium-reinforced cookware. In either case, titanium is a safe, inert metal. The nonstick surface of these products may be derived from silicone, a nonporous ceramic coating, titanium, or a combination thereof. As long as the coating isn't made with Teflon, nickel, or some other reactive metal, the products are considered safe. Glass containers are excellent to use when baking, as long as one uses a heat-tolerant glass such as Pyrex. CorningWare is also an excellent choice for baking foods in the oven. Neither Pyrex nor CorningWare can be placed on a range.

Utensils

The utensils that you stir or otherwise manipulate your food with while cooking are also important to consider. Nonstick coatings applied to utensils such as spatulas and spoons can leach out toxins, but if they are used properly and not overheated, this should not occur. As mentioned earlier, metal utensils can cause a scratching and scraping of surfaces, resulting in the flaking off of metals and/or coatings into your food. Wood and silicone products are nonabrasive and free from potentially toxic coatings. Although some people avoid using wooden spoons because they can become scratched and thus a potential breeding grounds for bacteria, if cleaned properly after each use they should last a very long time. We have used wooden spoons in our home for decades and have never had an issue with bacterial contamination.

Silicone is another product that seems to be a good choice for cooking utensils. Silicone is a synthetic polymer, an elastomer, manufactured by adding carbon and/or oxygen to the element silicon. Silicone can be formulated into a solid, liquid, or gel and has been used in many industries. In the medical industry, silicone has been used in implantable medical devices such as are utilized with joint replacements and breast implants and for injectable preparations. There have been many scientific papers written about potential negative outcomes in certain populations from the medical use of silicone,[27,28] but to date, there are no known health hazards associated with the use of silicone cookware. Products manufactured using silicone elastomers from Dow Corning can be placed in the freezer and, according to Dow Corning, are stable and safe up to over 500 degrees Fahrenheit. I prefer wood, but do find silicone cooking utensils to be very useful.

Cooking food

There are many different methods of cooking food, including baking, frying, sautéing, roasting, grilling, and microwaving. Why, I have a good friend who even created an "earth oven" in which she bakes bread and slow-cooks meats. If gas is used to cook food, whether on a range or in a conventional oven, one should always maintain good air ventilation in the kitchen, preferably with a fan that will vent the air to the outside. Electric ranges and ovens do not require the same ventilation.

Microwave ovens have been around for decades and were extraordinarily popular for a long time. Over the years though, disfavor has developed among health groups as the process of cooking food or even heating water with a microwave oven has become controversial. There are two main concerns with using a microwave to prepare food. One is the EMF radiation that is commonly emitted by the machine when it's operating. The other concern involves what the microwave actually does to the food in order to cook it.

When food is "nuked" in a microwave, a component of the electromagnetic spectrum with a wavelength just shorter than a radio wave transmits energy to water molecules within the food, causing them to vibrate. This vibration generates heat, which then passes into the surrounding food. Foods that contain more water will heat up more quickly than foods that are drier. This explains why heating foods in a microwave may result in uneven cooking. Portions of food not brought to proper temperature can raise health concerns as potential pathogenic bacteria may not be destroyed in the incompletely cooked cold spots.[29]

Microwaves affect the nutrients in food along with water, and scientists are still trying to understand the myriad of conflicting effects that microwaves can have on food. Some studies suggest minimal effect on the bioavailability of nutrients[30] while others show a clear nutrient degradation.[31] However, all cooking methods can affect the nutritional value of food.

A study designed by a Swiss researcher named Hans Hertel was the first to question the effects of microwave radiation on a food's nutritional value. His conclusions were that not only does microwave cooking change the nutrients in food, but that people who eat microwaved food have changes in their blood chemistry that show "deterioration." His research, published in *Search for Health* in 1992 and also in *Acres USA*, a publication dedicated to organic and sustainable farming, in the United States in 1994, went so far as to state that eating microwaved food causes cancer-type effects in the blood. He was quickly attacked by industry representatives and subsequently censored by the courts.[32]

In 1991, a woman was injected with blood serum that had been microwaved to bring it to proper temperature, and she died as a result. It has been determined that blood products, namely proteins in the blood, are somehow damaged or altered by microwaves.[33] I'm not suggesting that you could abruptly die from eating microwaved food, but it does seem clear that the proteins, fats, and other components of the food that you are eating can be "changed" by the microwaving process, just as the blood was "changed" in this unfortunate death. Although the alteration of food materials is poorly defined at this time, it is reasonable to assume that microwaving can affect digestibility and nutritional value.

Although perhaps less professionally scientific and certainly not peer- reviewed, my daughter did her own experiment for school in which she tried to grow potatoes in different sources of water to see if the type of water the potatoes were placed in would have an effect on their growth rate. Six different samples of water were tested, including distilled water, tap water, bottled water, pond water, filtered water, and water that had been previously microwaved for five minutes and then cooled back down to room temperature. Each category of water was tested three times by suspending an organic potato in each glass of water with toothpicks.

All of the potatoes grew except for those grown in the microwaved water samples. The three potatoes placed in the microwaved water all shriveled up and died! Why? I have no idea. If you enjoy the convenience of the microwave and are skeptical of its effect on food, this is an easy experiment that you can try at home. Make sure to use organic potatoes, because conventional varieties sold in markets may have been sprayed with a chemical agent to prevent sprouting.

To witness microwaved water's effect on the growth of a plant begs the question, What kind of effect does microwaved water have on the body? You may be convinced that even drinking the microwaved water of a hot beverage can have a detrimental effect on your health. Suddenly, even heating up a cup of coffee in the morning with a microwave oven doesn't seem like such a good idea.

Because of the results of our potato experiment, we tossed out the microwave three years ago and I can't say I've ever missed it.

Leftovers and food storage

Plastic wraps, aluminum foil, wax paper, plastic containers, and covered glass dishes are the most common short-term food storage materials. The goal of wrapping and storing material is, of course, to keep bacteria and mold from growing on the food's surface as well as to prevent food from drying out when stored on the counter, in the refrigerator, or in the freezer.

Food wraps

The most ubiquitous wrap in the kitchen is plastic wrap. Saran Wrap was accidentally discovered in 1933 at the Dow Chemical Company by a lab technician working to develop a new dry-cleaning product. The material created was initially turned into a liquid spray used on U.S. fighter planes and on automobile upholstery. Dow later named the product Saran and conducted further development to make the material appropriate for a kitchen wrap, removing the foul odor and clarifying the green color of the original material. Saran Wrap hit the commercial market in 1949 and the household market in 1953.

Saran Wrap was originally made of thin film polymers using polyvinylidene chloride (PVDC) containing phthalates, chemicals used to increase the wrap's flexibility. Unfortunately, it was discovered that phthalates can disrupt hormones when leached into food and thus are bad for one's health.[34] Phthalates have been linked to allergies, asthma[35,36] and abnormal sperm quality in adult men.[37]

Since 2006, almost all plastic wrap made in North America has been phthalate-free. But as phthalate was phased out, manufacturers introduced a new chemical: a low-density polyethylene (LDPE), which contains the plasticizer diethylhexyl adipate (DEHA). DEHA is another potential endocrine disruptor, and although there were concerns that it could cause cancer, the World Health Organization's International Agency for Research on Cancer concluded that there was not enough evidence to say that DEHA was carcinogenic.

According to Dow (the manufacturer of the Saran products), the company no longer uses plasticizers such as phthalates or DEHA in its products. In addition, it has taken chlorine out of the premium wrap formula in order to be more environmentally conscientious.

I don't recommend using Saran Wrap or any other plastic wrap directly on your food, especially fatty meats or cheeses, given that chemicals from plastic wrap more easily leach out into fats and oils. If you want to use plastic wrap, make sure your food has cooled before wrapping it. Then place a layer of unbleached parchment paper over the food and afterwards cover it with plastic wrap.

The plastics industry has a numbering system that denotes the type of chemical used to make each form of plastic. Labels on each plastic container are comprised of a number that is surrounded by three curved arrows that form a triangular shape. Some forms of plastic are safer; others are known to leach chemicals into food products. (A list of the industry's categories is found in Table 6.)

In general, products with a plastic code of 3 or V should be avoided, for both of these codes can indicate that the product contains polyvinylchloride. Plastics that are numbered 2 and 4 are less toxic than other plastics, given that they are composed of high-density and low- density polyethylene, respectively. Plastic wraps with the number 5 are composed of polypropylene, and are also generally considered safer to use.

Table 6. Categories of plastic

1 - PET (polyethylene terephthalate): Used to make plastic beverage bottles and some food packaging. This category of plastic may leach chemicals such as DEHA.

2 - HDPE (high-density polyethylene): Used in milk containers and plastic bags. This type is considered a safer form of plastic than the other categories.

3 - PVC (vinyl/polyvinyl chloride): Used to produce some food wraps. This category can potentially leach toxins.

4 - LDPE (low-density polyethylene): Found in shrink wraps, squeezable bottles, and plastic bags. Considered less toxic than other plastics.

5 -PP (polypropylene): Found in bottle tops, bags, and food wraps as well as yogurt and margarine containers. Considered one of the safest plastics.

6 - PS (polystyrene): Used for plastic utensils and Styrofoam packaging. May leach into food products.

7 - Others, such as LEXAN, polycarbonate and BPA (aka bisphenol A) Usually layered or mixed with other plastics.

Aluminum foil is a useful wrapping tool, but should be used carefully. As mentioned earlier, aluminum is a recognized neurotoxin and certain cancers and cases of infertility have been associated with aluminum toxicity. Best if you don't have aluminum foil directly contact your food, especially acidic foods such as cut tomatoes, tomato sauce, and citrus products like oranges and lemons. It has been shown that cooking foods in aluminum foil causes leaching of the metal into the food.[1] Instead, cover the food first with unbleached parchment paper and then, over that, wrap it with aluminum foil.

Wax paper is a common food wrap, but did you realize that most conventional brands of wax paper are coated with paraffin, a petroleum product? However, there are wax papers on the market that use soybean wax, which is nontoxic. If you prefer to use wax paper, it's best to opt for soybean-coated wax paper.

My personal choice for a food wrap is non-bleached parchment paper. Parchment paper is a wonderful food wrap, but be aware that there are two different varieties: bleached and non-bleached. The problem with bleached paper products in general—whether it's parchment paper, paper towels, or coffee filters—is that one of the byproducts of the bleaching process is dioxins, which are toxic. Dioxins can easily leach into food from paper products, so if you choose to wrap your food or bake your food in parchment paper, look for the unbleached variety. In fact, I'd recommend using only unbleached paper products in your kitchen, especially drip coffee filters. Hot coffee passing through a bleached filter can leach dioxins into the coffee, something that is easy to avoid as there are many unbleached coffee filters available for sale.

Food containers

Food containers are typically made of different varieties of hard plastic or glass. Tupperware is a common high-end brand of container that has been on the market for a long time. Tupperware states that since 2010 they have not sold items containing BPA, but that suggests their products manufactured before 2010 contained BPA. Regrettably, these products should probably be discarded. While BPA has been taken out of many plastics due to consumer demand, it has unfortunately been replaced in some instances with Bisphenol S (BPS) or Bisphenol F (BPF), both of which can affect the body's endocrine system, just as BPA does.[38] Studies show that BPS is found in 81% of random human blood samples tested.[39] Just as with water bottles, food storage containers that are labeled "BPA-free" may indeed be free of BPA free, but this doesn't mean they are BPS-free or BPF-free or safe from other potentially toxic additives and compounds.

Hard plastic containers will typically have a number on the bottom from 1 through 7 to denote the type of plastic. As detailed previously, the numbers 2, 4, and 5 are generally recognized as being safe for food and drink, whereas the numbers 3, 6, and 7 are considered a higher risk for toxicity. If you choose to use hard plastics for food storage, it's best not to store acidic or oily foods in them. Containers that are scratched up or badly worn should be discarded. Certainly do not microwave food in these containers or place them in the dishwasher on a high heat setting. You may even consider placing food items in unbleached parchment paper before placing them in a plastic container. This would provide a barrier between the food and the plastic, which may help a bit. Ideally though, I would recommend storing acidic and oily foods in glass containers.

Glass is the safest material to use for storing food. Glass is heavy and it can shatter if it is dropped, but it is inert and will not react with food. Prices for glass food storage containers have come down as the demand for them has increased. As mentioned earlier, make sure that the glass containers you use are not painted on the inside where the food is placed. If possible, try to obtain glass containers that are made in the United States and not imported from China. Glass from China has been found to contain lead and/or cadmium,[40,41] especially if there is paint or enamel on the product. Pyrex and Anchor Hocking are two excellent American manufacturers. Glass containers may be used with plastic lids or may be covered with a plastic wrap or aluminum foil if the food doesn't come into contact with the covering. Otherwise, use a larger container. Glass Mason jars are also an excellent, inexpensive way to store leftover food.

So, in summary, pay attention to the cookware and food storage items you use in your kitchen. If you are cooking on a nonstick pan coated with Teflon or a similar product, consider switching to a safer alternative such as anodized aluminum or cast iron. If your favorite pan is scratched, scraped, or worn, bite the bullet and toss it. There are many different brands of safe pots and pans on the market, but it is best to stay away from non-anodized aluminum, copper, and coated surfaces such as Teflon. Cooking utensils do not typically get as hot as a frying pan or cooking pot. Given this, wood and silicone utensils seem to be the safest materials at present to cook with.

Try and take the extra time necessary to cook with electricity or gas and forget the microwave. The microwave has poorly understood effects on food, and I wouldn't use it even to heat up plain water. Better to take a few minutes out of your busy day to prepare your food in an oven or on a range. If you are using plastic wrap, plastic containers, or aluminum foil, consider adding a layer of unbleached parchment paper over the food before covering it with your preferred product.

These simple alterations to your cooking and food storage practices will significantly reduce your exposure to all kinds of potential toxins in the kitchen.

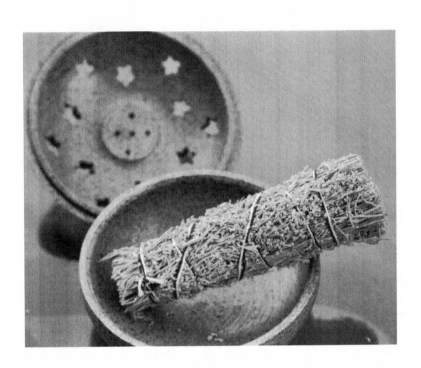

Chapter 6
HOME CLEANING

The house cleaning industry is enormous and growing all of the time. Depending on your cleaning habits, this chapter may help you relax by giving you permission to ease up on your cleaning. Or, it could help you focus your effort on what's really important when cleaning your home.

If you believe that everything in your home needs to be sanitized and sterilized with antibacterial sprays and wipes, consider this to be the result of successful indoctrination by the American Cleaning Institute, an organization that will tell you that everything everywhere needs to be cleaned by one or more of their industry's products. In fact, there is plenty of evidence to support the idea that having bacteria in your home is important and in fact necessary for a properly functioning immune system.[1]

Researchers have observed that children who grow up on farms, playing with animals and living amidst the soil, are frequently much healthier and have stronger immune systems than children who grow up in sterilized quarters that are frequently sprayed and wiped down with antibacterial agents.[2] The microbiome that protects your body from pathogenic bacteria is not only on your skin surface and in your gut, but also throughout your home. We are dropping bacteria and picking up bacteria all of the time,[3] which is a good thing for our overall health. Good hygiene and proper sanitation to remove waste from the home is extraordinarily important to prevent disease, but a home can be too clean, which can also be damaging to the immune system. This "hygiene hypothesis" was introduced into the scientific literature in 1989.[4]

Product regulation and safety

The safety of cleaning supplies has undergone progressive disclosure over the years. Before 2009, the only protection offered to consumers was through the Federal Hazardous Substances Act (FHSA), which requires labeling on household products that the government considers to be potentially hazardous to one's health. This act only considers products that are toxic, corrosive, flammable, combustible, or potentially explosive to be dangerous. If a product has one of these characteristics, packaging needs to be affixed with a caution label. Products are labeled irritants if they can cause serious injury to a part of the body that is exposed to the product. A sensitizer label is affixed to those products one can quickly become allergic to upon a second exposure. The FHSA allows the Consumer Product Safety Commission to ban products that it considers to be too dangerous for household use. Whereas this act provides oversight for specific categories of hazardous material, regulations do not provide oversight for products that are more insidiously toxic, meaning those materials that can cause chronic disease, including cancer.

In 2009, the Household Product Labeling Act went into effect, requiring companies to list ingredients contained within cleaning products, air fresheners, and paint on the products' packaging. Unfortunately, though, this act does not require that all product ingredients be disclosed on a product's label. Fragrances, dyes, and ingredients that make up less than 1% of a product's weight need not be listed, as these are considered to be proprietary, confidential formulae.

The determination of a product's toxicity takes into account parameters such as the concentration of chemicals, the route of potential exposure, and the duration of exposure. Toxicologists determine if there are potentially harmful effects to an individual given the expected concentration and typical duration of exposure during intended use of the product. With so many chemicals that can be dangerous if used improperly, the question is, how often do we stray from printed directions for intended use? If, for example, you are using a floor cleaner and the instructions on the cleaner label specify to dilute one capful of the product into a gallon of water, what will the typical user do when in a hurry or feeling lazy? If there is a bad carpet stain, one might try to pour a little bit of a cleaning solution directly onto the stain instead of diluting the product, believing that this will make the product work better. Directions may also specify to wear nitrile gloves during application, but one may choose to use the product with latex gloves or possibly without any gloves. Frequently, the use of home cleaning products in a method other than intended may bring on negative health consequences. Many household cleaning products can cause a broad spectrum of negative health effects, including endocrine disruption.[5]

Words on labeling specify the degree of concern one should have when handling these products. *CAUTION* or *WARNING* is used on a label if the product may cause what is considered to be a mild hazard to your health. The most common entry points for these types of chemicals are through the skin and lungs,[6] so those are the two organ systems that need to be considered when using these cleaning products. Many laundry detergents, disinfectants, all-purpose cleaners, and dishwasher detergents fall into this category. A *CAUTION* label on a dishwasher detergent gives one pause when considering that many dishwashers leave tiny particles of detergent on plates, cups, and glasses after the rinse cycle completes.

Products labeled *DANGER* are potentially more toxic than those with the *CAUTION* or *WARNING* label. These products are typically used to clean specialty items, such as ovens and clogged drains. Products with a *DANGER* label can cause serious damage if they make direct contact with the skin and eyes by accidental splashing. Flammable products also require the *DANGER* label if they have the potential to ignite when exposed to an open flame. The *POISON* label is reserved for the most dangerous category of toxins and indicates that accidental exposure can cause severe medical effects, including death. If lye is swallowed, for example, a severe chemical burn of the esophagus will ensue and the lining of the esophagus will slough off. As the body tries to repair the damage, extensive scarring will develop. The esophagus, once distensible, will become a very narrow and rigid tube, severely limiting the ability of food and liquids to pass through. As if that weren't bad enough, cancer of the esophagus can then develop.

Do you know where your nearest poison control center is? If not, take a moment to look this up. Whereas many household cleaning products can be washed down the drain or flushed down the toilet, not all products are biodegradable. Before using a new product, check the label to see if there are any special instructions for the product's disposal. Improper disposal can cause environmental damage. Please, don't throw a toxic cleaner into the trash or down the drain if there are directions telling you to do otherwise.

Surfactants, disinfectants, and pH

Cleaning materials take advantage of many different chemical interactions to help them work. The most common mechanisms for household cleaning include the use of surfactants, disinfectants, and pH manipulation.

Surfactants are chemicals that break the surface tension of water. Surface tension is a characteristic of water that results from the underlying attraction that water molecules have to one another. The property of surface tension explains why a droplet of water will form a bead when placed on a flat surface such as a countertop. Surfactant molecules slip in between individual water molecules, getting in the way of the attractive forces of the tiny water magnets, thereby breaking the surface tension. As a result, instead of beading, water will spread out on materials and surfaces, effectively making the water "wetter."

Surfactants, like water, have two poles. But, instead of these two poles being opposite charges, one end of the molecule is hydrophilic, meaning that it is attracted to water, while the other pole is hydrophobic, meaning that it is repelled by water. The hydrophilic portion of the molecule can have different characteristics, depending on whether or not it has a charge.

Soap is a surfactant. The cleansing characteristics of soap stem from the differing chemical characteristics of its molecule's poles. Soaps with either a negatively charged or uncharged hydrophilic component are referred to as anionic and nonionic, respectively, whereas surfactants with a positive charge are referred to as cationic. The hydrophilic portion of the molecule in soap is typically made from a molecule containing either sodium or potassium. The soaps made with sodium are harder and are used to form bars of soap, whereas the potassium soaps are softer and are more commonly used to make liquid soaps. The hydrophobic portion of a surfactant molecule is composed of a chain of carbon atoms surrounded by hydrogen atoms, similar to a fatty acid, one of the components of a fat molecule. Soaps and other surfactants were originally produced by taking this fatty acid component from plant and animal fats and oils.

If your water is "hard" (containing minerals such as calcium, magnesium, iron, or manganese), soap molecules will bond to the minerals and produce an insoluble precipitate, commonly referred to as soap scum, which will streak and smear on surfaces. As precipitates form, more and more soap molecules are removed from the cleaning solution, decreasing the effectiveness of the soap. Metals causing precipitation most commonly originate from the water source itself, but can also arise from materials being cleaned. For example, if you have clothing caked with mud, washing it with regular soap will cause precipitates to form as the soap binds to metals in the soil, even if the water itself is free of metals. The first laundry soaps in the 1920s allowed precipitants to form and as a result, clothes that were laundered back then didn't look too clean.

Detergents differ from basic soap in that they are commonly composed of more than one surfactant and usually contain other ingredients to aid in cleaning. In the US, the first synthetic detergents were produced in the early 1930s. Since then, numerous revisions have occurred and the complexity of detergents has dramatically increased over time. Detergents now contain ingredients such as "builders," and are formulated to be less reactive to metals than ordinary soap and therefore don't precipitate as easily. Builders help surfactants penetrate deeply into fabrics to get clothing cleaner. Chemicals derived from petroleum (i.e. petrochemicals) are now commonly used as a source of fatty acids in lieu of animal and plant fats to create components of the detergent mixture.

The pH measurement indicates the extent to which a solution is either acidic or alkaline. Acidic solutions have free hydrogen atoms (H+) within them which are able to react with negatively charged ions, compounds, or molecules. A basic or alkaline product contains free hydroxide (OH-) ions which can react with positively charged particles. The pH scale ranges from 1 to 14. A solution with a pH of 7 is neutral, containing equal numbers of H+ and OH- ions. Pure water, the molecule H_2O, can also be written as HOH and dissociates into both a H+ ion and a OH- ion, yielding a pH of 7.

Cleaning products take advantage of pH and may be either acidic or alkaline. Acids are better able to remove hard water, mineral deposits, and rust stains. They are also useful to kill mold and mildew, and are therefore very useful in the bathroom. Rust-removing solutions, toilet bowl cleaners, and tub and tile cleansers are all acidic cleaning solutions. Acidic foods, such as lemons and limes, oranges, coffee, and cola can also be used as cleaning agents in some situations, for example, to remove a rust stain. Alkaline solutions help remove fats and oils from surfaces. Most hand soaps are mildly alkaline so they can effectively remove oils from skin. Markedly alkaline materials can be very dangerous, even more dangerous than acidic solutions, if accidentally swallowed or spilled on the skin. Alkaline solutions can kill all sorts of microorganisms, including bacteria, molds, mildew, and viruses. Bleach is alkaline, with a pH of 12.5. Detergents, all-purpose cleaners, and oven cleaners are all typically alkaline.

In general, cleaning products are formulated with a pH that will offer the product its maximum cleaning efficacy. The scale below illustrates the levels of several common foods and cleaners (Figure 3).

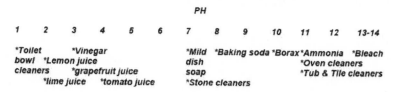

Figure 3. pH of common house hold cleansers

PH

| 1 | 2 | 3 | 4 | 5 | 6 | 7 | 8 | 9 | 10 | 11 | 12 | 13-14 |

Toilet   *Vinegar*   *Mild*   *Baking soda* *Borax* *Ammonia*   *Bleach*
bowl   *Lemon juice*   *dish*   *Oven cleaners*
cleaners   *grapefruit juice*   *soap*   *Tub & Tile cleaners*
        lime juice   *tomato juice*   *Stone cleaners*

Kitchen care

Kitchen cleaning is the most frequent chore in the typical home. Countertops are wiped down several times a day, the floor is mopped at least weekly, and dishes and glassware are washed several times a day. It is important to be diligent and to make sure that all food preparation surfaces, utensils, and eating surfaces are properly cleansed so that food isn't contaminated prior to eating or during storage.

Countertop cleaning

There are many counter sprays on the market designed to clean and sanitize. The Environmental Working Group website is a wonderful resource and contains information about most of the products in the marketplace and grades them from A to F. Look up the product you like to use and see if you are happy with its grade. If not, look for alternatives. Consider homemade solutions.

For a countertop cleaner, fill a one-quart spray bottle with warm water and four tablespoons of baking soda. You will have enough counter spray to last a year. Add fragrance by mixing in a few drops of essential oil. This solution won't sterilize your countertop, but it will clean it sufficiently. Baking soda is an excellent natural scouring agent and can also be used to clean your sink instead of using a more toxic alternative.

To create a healthier cleanser that will sanitize your countertop, make a disinfecting countertop spray by filling a one-quart spray bottle with one cup of vinegar, a few tablespoons of lemon juice, and a few drops of an essential oil, and then fill it up with warm water. This solution will kill almost all of the bacteria on your countertop.

Alternatively, if you are a bleach fan, you can fill a quart spray bottle with water and add 3/4 tsp of bleach. This will yield a solution that is 200 ppm, perfectly adequate for sanitizing your countertops and kitchen equipment. After you spray it on a surface, let it air dry. This will allow the bleach to kill the bacteria and any other potential pathogens. This mixture will lose its potency over time, so after three months, add another 3/4 tsp of bleach to strengthen the solution again.

It is usually unnecessary to sterilize your countertops. Try less toxic mixtures and leave the bleach spray for special occasions when someone in the house is sick or if the countertop becomes particularly soiled. Studies have shown that weekly use of bleach in the home is associated with more frequent illnesses in children. A recent study from Belgium has shown an association with bleach and a 20% increase in the flu, a 35% increase in tonsillitis, and an 18% increase in other infections in children between the ages of 6 and 12.[7] Predisposing yourself and your children to increased risk of disease makes no sense if you are trying to sterilize your countertops in order to keep yourself and your children from getting sick. Some scientists think that gases evaporating from the bleach cause irritation of the airways and lungs, resulting in inflammation and a greater susceptibility to disease, including asthma.[8]

Although the emphasis on kitchen cleaning is usually on soaps and other cleaning agents, high-quality cleansing rags, scouring pads, and brushes are equally, if not more important. It is important to use clean, dry dish rags when you wipe your countertop. After each use, rags should be rinsed of food debris and placed on a rack or over a rail to dry. If cleaning rags aren't given time to dry, they will stay moist, which will then allow bacteria and fungi to grow on their surface. Wiping the kitchen counter down with a damp rag that has bacteria growing on it will spread bacteria onto the surface of your counter, exactly the opposite of your intention. Some companies infuse their cleaning cloths with silver fibers or nanoparticles. These cloths are expensive, but the silver will inhibit the growth of microorganisms, providing extra protection against bacterial colonization.[9] However, if you decide to try this technology, be aware that silver nanoparticles added to textiles and clothing items have been shown to migrate out of the fabric during washing, ending up in the environment through wastewater.[10]

Dishwasher liquids and powders

Did you know that the number-one cause of household poisoning is from dish detergent? Because of its alkalinity, dish detergent will cause severe burns in the mouth, throat, and esophagus if accidentally swallowed. As with lye, as the burns heal, they form scars that narrow the passageway. Swallowing dish detergent may even be fatal. If you have small children in your home, you most likely have safety latches on the kitchen cabinets containing cleansers. Another option, though, is to use an organic detergent, a healthier choice. Check the EWG website to find a preferable brand with an A or B rating. Making your own dish soap is a bit more involved than making a counter spray, but is certainly doable. There are many websites available that will provide homemade dishwasher soap recipes. If you have the time, go for it! If not, opt for a detergent that has fewer chemicals and no dyes or fragrance. Remove all food debris from your dishes and silverware before placing the items into the dishwasher. It doesn't take much time and if you do, you don't have to worry about getting a super- aggressive dishwasher cleanser to dissolve and destroy all of the bits of food that have encrusted your dishes.

When first writing this book, I had a section dedicated to eliminating "antibacterial" dishwashing liquids and soaps from your home. Many research papers have warned of the endocrine-disrupting characteristics of triclosan, a synthetic antimicrobial agent added to these soaps. Since then, the FDA has banned triclosan and other antibacterial additives for use in soaps, so it is no longer a choice in the US.[11]

Triclosan is a bioaccumulating particle[12] that may cause a weakened immune system by damaging the microbiome, especially if you accidentally ingest traces of it.[13]

As many dishwashers don't remove all of the soapy residue from the plates, glasses, and silverware, chances are, many of us have ingested small amounts of dish detergent over the years. It really is a good idea to look for a less toxic dish detergent.

Oven cleaner

Cleaning the oven is an infrequent and potentially dangerous task. Many people have gotten sick or injured using these products. There are typically three methods to choose from when cleaning the oven: toxic commercial products, the self-cleaning function offered on many ovens, and safer, natural products without harsh chemicals, which may or may not require elbow grease.

Conventional oven cleaners can be very toxic and as mentioned on their labeling, can be fatal if swallowed. Oven cleaners are typically very alkaline. If swallowed, these chemicals will cause severe chemical burns of the gastrointestinal tract. If you have children at home, having a toxic oven cleaner in an accessible cabinet is not a good idea. To prevent accidents, make sure to lock the cabinet or place the product somewhere where children and animals will not have access to it.

Self-cleaning ovens do a great job destroying the crud that builds up on the interior of the oven, and are very convenient. The accompanying instructions typically recommend that you open windows and doors and turn on ceiling fans and vents whenever you use the self-cleaning feature, as burnt drippings accumulated on the oven bottom can produce carbon monoxide when incinerated during the cleaning process. If the walls of the self-cleaning oven are treated with a nonstick coating such as Teflon, I'd do all of that, plus then get yourself, your family, and your pets out of the house until the process has been over for a couple of hours. Many new technologies, however, are being developed to create nonstick surfaces that do not produce toxic fumes. So, when purchasing a new oven, inquire about the self-cleaning feature and investigate the materials that line the oven's interior.

Although it takes more time, an oven can be cleaned manually with a pumice stick and water. Before attempting to manually clean your oven, check your owner's manual to make sure the stone won't damage the interior. Alternatively, you can use the usual kitchen staples to try and clean it, including baking soda, vinegar, and citrus, such as lemon juice or lemon peel. You can make a solution of baking soda and water and spray the inside of the oven and either let the mixture sit on the gunk overnight or turn the oven on low for an hour. Because of its alkalinity, the baking soda should cause a saponification effect on the grease which should then allow the mess to be wiped off after the oven cools down. You can also spray some white vinegar on the oven surface after applying baking soda to further loosen the burnt-on debris. Placing lemon or orange peels in a shallow pan, covering them with water, and then baking them in the oven for twenty minutes may also help dissolve burnt-on material. Let the oven cool before wiping the surfaces down so as not to burn yourself.

Once you get used to using edible cleaning agents in the kitchen, such as vinegar, baking soda, and lemon juice, you may question why you hadn't thought to use these materials before.

Bathroom

Most people wear latex gloves to protect their hands while cleaning the bathroom, but it's usually to protect themselves from the stuff on the floor rather than from the cleaning materials themselves. Bathroom cleansers are typically very harsh agents designed to kill all types of bacteria, viruses, and molds. In addition to possibly causing skin reactions, bathroom cleaners can aerosolize and cause respiratory irritation if used with inadequate ventilation. There are specialized cleaners designed for the floor, countertop, mirrors, and porcelain surfaces such as the sink, tub, shower stall, and toilet.

With some basic good hygiene, bathroom cleaning can be less arduous. For instance, before flushing the toilet, close the lid. Although you can't see it with your eyes, bacteria are present in large concentrations in the toilet water, even after flushing, and water vapor with accompanying bacteria can aerosolize and cover bathroom surfaces when the toilet is flushed with the lid up.[14]

There are so many toilet bowl cleansers in the market. Research the EWG website and look up the cleanser you use and see how it rates. Stronger cleansers do not need to be used for weekly or biweekly maintenance cleaning, but should be reserved for a few times a year, such as if hard water stains develop. For routine maintenance, an abrasive such as baking soda can be used to remove particulates, followed by vinegar, an effective disinfectant. Adding a few drops of any essential oil into the baking soda before adding it to the water can provide fragrance. First, scour the toilet bowl with baking soda mixture and then flush. Afterwards, add white vinegar to the toilet bowl and scour. If the toilet has a hard water ring or is stained, let the vinegar sit in the toilet for an hour before scouring. The acidic quality of vinegar should be effective at removing hard water rings and stains, but it will need time to react chemically with the deposits. It is important to flush the toilet after scouring with baking soda and before adding vinegar. If not, the alkaline baking soda will neutralize the acidic vinegar, rendering it ineffective at disinfecting. If this process doesn't clean satisfactorily, a 1/4 cup of bleach or a commercial product can be poured into the toilet, but remember to turn on the fan, open the windows, and put on a pair of rubber gloves before using a brush to clean the bowl.

Drop-ins designed for the toilet are unnecessary. These products turn the water an unnatural shade of blue, which can prevent one from observing the state of their excrement. It is important, for example, to recognize if there is a small amount of blood in the urine or stool, both important indicators of a medical problem. If the toilet is manually cleaned each week with a scouring brush and a cleaner, there shouldn't be any odor emanating from your toilet.

The bathroom has the potential for developing mold and mildew from ordinary, everyday use. These forms of fungus require water for growth. As mold grows, it quickly produces spores which can then aerosolize and spread to the other dampened surfaces. If steps are taken to prevent mold from growing in the first place, there will be less of a reason to use mold and mildew cleaners in the bathroom.

The first thing to consider is that mold and mildew need moist or wet surfaces to grow on. Search the bathroom for hidden sources of moisture. Shower curtains should be pulled closed after use so water doesn't accumulate within the folds. When taking a shower, either open a window or turn on the vent to circulate air so humidity doesn't build up and leave a film of water vapor on all of the bathroom surfaces. Opening the bathroom window not only reduces indoor humidity, but also allows more light into the room, which hinders some forms of mold growth. Spread dampened towels out on a rack to air-dry quickly. If a fabric, such as a towel, remains damp for extended periods of time, mold and mildew will make it their newest home. To further reduce humidity, wipe up puddles of water that may splash onto the countertop or floor. If, despite these practices, humidity remains a problem, placing a dehumidifier in the bathroom will solve the problem.

Before cleaning porcelain surfaces, look up your tub and tile cleaner on the EWG website to see how it rates. Alternatively, porcelain fixtures can usually be cleaned satisfactorily with warm water and a mild abrasive, such as baking soda, followed by a solution containing vinegar or a simple soap. Vinegar will help dissolve soap scum. The pipes draining porcelain fixtures should also be cleaned every month or two, but instead of using a toxic chemical, try first pouring down 1/2 cup of baking soda along with some water down the drain. Then, follow the baking soda with 1/2 cup of white vinegar. Let the mixture stand in the drain for five or ten minutes while you bring a few cups of water to a boil in the kitchen. Pour boiling water down the drain to flush out any clogged material. This technique will help remove any persistent odor coming from your drain. If odors persist, cover the drain with a plug or stopper when it is not in use. This may be necessary when living in an apartment building. Closing or covering the drain will certainly prevent odors from permeating your bathroom and home and will also help prevent unwanted bugs, such as roaches, from entering.

Accessories in the bathroom should be cleaned regularly. Wipe surfaces that people touch frequently, such as the toilet handle, door knobs, water faucets, and the tub/shower knobs. Shower liners need to be washed periodically and then air-dried promptly to prevent mildew. Most liners can be placed into the washing machine or you can scrub the liner with a cleaning solution and a gloved hand. Tea tree oil, an essential oil with a pleasing scent, can be added to your natural bathroom cleanser as a disinfectant. Tea tree oil has antibacterial, anti-fungal, and antiviral properties,[15] so it will safely sanitize your bathroom surfaces without toxicity.

A sanitizing solution can also be created by diluting bleach into water. In order to disinfect bathroom surfaces with bleach, dilute the bleach in a solution that is approximately 500 ppm, more concentrated than what is normally used for kitchen countertops. This dilution can be achieved by adding 2 tsp of bleach into 1 quart of water. Be cautious not to mix a bleach disinfectant with your other homemade cleaning solutions. If bleach and vinegar are mixed together, they'll release a dangerous chlorine gas.

Bleach will sanitize a surface that is already clean, so save sanitation for the last step. Spray the bleach solution onto surfaces and then let it sit for at least ten minutes in order for the solution to be effective. Provided your bathroom has good ventilation, surfaces can be left to air-dry.

A bleach solution can also be used with a soft bristled brush to clean bathroom grout. Studies have shown that dilute bleach will lose up to 50% of its strength within thirty days if it is stored in a container other than a closed, brown container.[16] So if you choose to disinfect your bathroom with bleach, make up a new solution monthly.

The arrangement of toiletries around the bathroom sink can help everyone stay healthy or allow everyone to share viruses. It is a good idea for each member of the household to have their own drinking cup. Some households choose paper cups in the bathroom. Toothbrushes should also be kept separate from each other and either stored in each person's drinking vessel or in a toothbrush stand where the brushes don't contact each other. In that way, potential bacteria on one brush won't transmit to the others.

Mold and mildew

As mentioned earlier, mold and mildew can grow anywhere there is excessive, prolonged moisture. If you have mold or mildew growing in an area of your house that doesn't have an obvious link to a water source, consider the growth as a red flag, and address it. If the underlying source of water is not eliminated, mold will grow back after you attempt to eradicate it.

Unintended moisture may occur from a leaky pipe, a leaky roof or window, or be secondary to an exterior drainage problem. If water is accumulating next to the house exterior and getting absorbed by the foundation and walls, mold growth can appear in the basement and ground-level rooms. Excessive moisture can also arise because of temperature fluctuations within the home, especially if ductwork and walls are improperly insulated. As warm air hits cooler air, water vapor in the warmer air condenses, causing moisture. If an area in the home becomes water-saturated, dry it out within twenty-four hours to prevent mold and mildew growth. Fungal spores are ubiquitous, so even if you haven't previously had a mold problem, spores will find their way to damp areas and set up colonies.

Mold and mildew need to be cleaned up and removed. Fungal spores can cause lung disease in certain people, so if you clean up the mold yourself, wear an N-95 particulate respirator. These masks cover your nose and mouth and will protect you from inhaling mold spores. They are inexpensive and can be purchased at any hardware store or big-box store. It would be a good idea to also wear goggles and gloves to prevent the mold spores from getting into your eyes and to protect your skin from the cleaning solution.

There are homemade cleaning solutions that will effectively kill mold and mildew. Initially, mix 2 tablespoons of baking soda into 8 oz of water and spray the solution on the moldy surface. You can also sprinkle dry baking soda on the surface and allow it to react with the mold without water. In general, porous surfaces that become moldy need to be thrown out because there is no way to kill all of the mold growing within the pores. But if you have a porous surface you can't dispose of, sprinkling baking soda onto the moldy area may help, as the baking soda dust will permeate the surface and enter the porous surfaces. Five or ten minutes after applying the baking soda, wipe the surface clean.

If mold persists, spray or pour vinegar, either apple cider vinegar or white vinegar, on to the residual mold and scrub it with a brush. Vinegar will usually eliminate the mold and mildew by itself, but pretreatment with baking soda will increase the vinegar's effectiveness. If the mold grows back or isn't successfully eliminated following this treatment, try applying solutions of either borax or hydrogen peroxide and waiting ten minutes before attempting to scrub the mold off. Hydrogen peroxide can be safely used on almost any surface. When using hydrogen peroxide, though, do a spot test on an inconspicuous piece of the material being treated to make sure no discoloration occurs.

If none of these solutions are effective at removing the mold, try bleach. Open up the windows, turn on a fan, and then mix 1/4 cup of bleach in a quart of water. Wipe or spray the solution on the mold and scrub it with a brush. When finished, dry the surface.

If you have an area with recurrent mold buildup, or a larger area involved, it would be best to call a professional service to eradicate it. Some forms of mold produce toxins, so all mold needs to be removed.

All-purpose cleaners

When choosing a general household cleaner, most consumers are looking for a product that can cut through grease, remove stains, eliminate mildew and mineral deposits, and kill bacteria. Many desire a "spotless" home, rather than a healthy home. Weekly cleaning with antibacterial solutions and cleansers containing bleach is usually unnecessary and may harm your health not only by causing respiratory irritation, but also through the elimination of helpful bacteria that form your external microbiome.[17]

So, when considering which all-purpose cleanser to use in your home, think first about what needs to be cleaned in order to maintain a healthy home environment. Maximize the clean "look" without compromising your health. When looking at rating systems, consider the source. For example, a common national brand all-purpose cleaning product received a top rating of 4/4 stars on a popular home consumer reference website due to this cleaner's ability to remove dried dirt stains from stainless steel, countertops, and painted walls, though it left behind light streaks and smears. In addition, this product could be used on mirrors and appliances as well as on sealed granite. Sounds good, right? This same product received an F rating on the EWG website. Although the product cleans well, the EWG website reports that the chemicals in this particular product can damage the nervous and respiratory systems. Consider creating your own cleaning solutions at home. It is not as difficult as it may sound.

pH

Neutralizing pH is a useful strategy in household cleaning. Dirt and grime are acidic and more easily cleaned with an alkaline material such as baking soda, whereas alkaline stains are more easily removed with an acidic material such as lemon juice. Edible kitchen staples such as vinegar, lemon juice, and baking soda can clean most everything in your house. Adding an essential oil to the mixture will provide fragrance.

You can use a pH test strip to measure the commercial products that you ordinarily use. Then, try to replicate the pH with your own ingredients. For example, in place of bleach, which is a strong alkaline, substitute baking soda, which is also alkaline, although not as strong. Toilet bowl cleaners are typically strongly acidic, but substituting vinegar and even adding a few squirts of lemon juice to the solution will decrease the pH of the water in order to effectively clean the toilet bowl.

For a general household cleaner, mix undiluted white vinegar and coarse salt together. The vinegar will cut grease, remove mildew and odors, clean stains, and remove wax build-up. The salt will act as an abrasive to help further clean hard surfaces. As with any cleaner, test the solution on an inconspicuous spot to make sure it doesn't damage the finish of the surface. A solution created by mixing one tablespoon of baking soda in one cup of water can also be used to scour surfaces. Below is a list of household staples with their associated pH levels and potential uses (Table 7).

Table 7. pH of common household staples

pH 2: Lemon juice – kills most household bacteria.

pH 3: White vinegar – cuts grease, removes mildew, odors, stains, and wax build-up.

pH 4-5: Hydrogen peroxide (pH varies but this is the range for dilute products 3-10%) - disinfectant, stain remover

pH 4.0-7.0: Cornstarch – can be used to clean windows, polish furniture, or as shampoo.

pH 5.5: Isopropyl alcohol – disinfectant. pH 7.0: Water - universal solvent

pH 8: Baking soda – scours, softens water, deodorizes, and cleans; good for refrigerator.

pH 8.9: Castille soap - Cleans, natural insecticide

pH 10: Borax – cleans, deodorizes, disinfects; can be used to clean walls and floors.

Vinegar and bleach

Be mindful using vinegar. As mentioned earlier, don't mix vinegar or any ammonia-based cleaner with bleach. These chemicals will react with each other when mixed and produce a dangerous toxic gas. Mixing vinegar with hydrogen peroxide will create a strong, very corrosive compound called peracetic acid, which has powerful antimicrobial properties.[18] If you want to experiment with this acid as a disinfectant, be careful where you use it. Open windows and make sure there is good ventilation, because the fumes from this acid are corrosive to the lining of the respiratory tract. In addition, wear nitrile gloves to protect your skin. Vinegar and baking soda also need to be used separately or sequentially, but not together. If these two agents are mixed together, the acidic nature of the vinegar will be neutralized by the alkalinity of the baking soda. Adding water to any cleaning solution, including vinegar, is almost always safe, but it will reduce the cleaner's effectiveness by reducing the pH of alkaline materials and raising the pH of acidic materials.

Many who make their own cleansers at home avoid bleach, which contains a chemical called sodium hypochlorite. Sodium hypochlorite is strongly alkaline, but is not a surfactant and not a cleanser. Bleach can be used, however, as a disinfectant after cleaning. It can be used to sterilize a specific area, but as always, use it in a well-ventilated area while wearing protective gloves and eyewear.

Bleach solutions for home use are typically in lower concentrations, between 3-8%. Even in lower concentrations, liquid bleach can react with your skin and cause inflammation, referred to as an irritant contact dermatitis.[19] The gas evaporating from the solution can react with the covering of your eyes, the mucosal lining of your nose, and your respiratory tract.[20] In 2012, bleach was been labeled an asthmagen by the Association of Occupational and Environmental Clinics, meaning that not only can it cause an asthma attack in someone with pre-existing asthma, it can also cause someone to develop asthma.[21] It would be best for the overall health of your household if you could wean yourself off from using bleach for your all-purpose cleaning and choose less toxic alternatives. If you do choose to use it on occasion, do not mix it with other household chemicals, especially vinegar and rubbing alcohol.

Cleaning tools

Cleaning tools can be just as important a choice as the cleaning solutions themselves. A good cloth will allow you to clean with less cleaning solution, and in some cases, with only water. Microfiber cloths attract dirt and other materials to thousands of tiny protrusions arising from the cloth's surface, which significantly increase the surface area of the cloth and offer a three- dimensional surface for dust and dirt to accumulate on. In comparison, a cotton cloth with a two-dimensional cleaning surface is much less efficient.

Another versatile cleaning tool is a pumice stone. Pumice is a soft mineral which has been used as a cleaning agent for millennia. It has even been used to clean the skin and remove calluses from the feet. A pumice stone or stick purchased at a local hardware store can be used to clean all sorts of scratch-resistant surfaces, such as ovens, oven racks, barbecues, and grills, and can also be used to remove rust and debris from pipes. A pumice stick can also be used to clean porcelain surfaces, including toilet bowls. You will no doubt find many uses for a pumice stone once you have one.

Glass cleaners

These sprays are designed for hard-surface cleaning, such as glass and tile. According to the Windex website, all but two of their products contain detergents, solvents, fragrance, Ammonia-D, and alcohol. According to the EWG, Windex also contains chemicals, such as hexoxyethanol and ammonium hydroxide, which is a respiratory irritant and can damage eyesight.[22] Homemade glass-cleaning solutions offer a safer alternative. A quick Google search will present you with many options for non-toxic homemade glass cleaning solutions. The simplest concoction is mixing vinegar and water and wiping the solution off with newsprint, or better yet, a microfiber cloth. Other ingredients such as lemon juice, corn starch, baking soda, or essential oils for fragrance can also be added. It may take a bit of research initially, but once you have your own homemade recipe, you'll find that it is not only less expensive than buying a commercial product, it is less toxic and will work just as well.

Floor care

Pine-Sol was invented in 1929 and is now produced and distributed by the Clorox company. Did you know that Pine-Sol is the biggest selling household cleaner in the world? On the Pine-Sol website, you can find a list of ingredients for their original multi-surface cleaner:

Water
C10-12 Alcohol Ethoxylates
Caramel
Fragrance
Glycolic Acid
Methylisothiazolinone
Octylisothiazolinone
Sodium C14-17 Sec-Alkyl Sulfonate

As of 2016, according to the company's FAQ sheet, pine oil is no longer an ingredient in Pine-Sol due to its increasing cost and limited supply.[23] As with all labeling, only ingredients that make up 1% or more of the product are listed. Ingredients excluded from the list would also include byproducts and contaminants. At the risk of being too repetitive, you can easily make your own floor cleaner for less money and with fewer chemicals. Actually, all you really need to clean hardwood floors is a mop, water, and vinegar. If you choose, adding pure Castille soap and essential oil will make a fragrant, soapy cleaning solution that may be more to your liking than merely vinegar and water.

Another popular hard-flooring surface cleaner is the Swiffer. This mopping system uses less liquid to clean than a traditional mop and is very convenient, but using a mop and a homemade floor-cleaning solution is even safer and certainly less expensive.

Carpeting requires maintenance. Aside from regularly vacuuming to remove accumulated dust and debris, carpets can develop odors. The chemicals used in powders designed to be sprinkled on carpets to make them smell fresh are a big unknown. Carpet Fresh, made by the company that produces the lubricant WD-40, is one such product. The proprietary ingredients are top-secret. People and animals may experience itchy eyes and sinus symptoms after walking into a home that has been treated with a fragrant carpet powder, as these products can cause irritation and allergic reactions.[24]

Baking soda will remove carpet odors without using unknown chemicals and fragrances. Sprinkle baking soda on your carpet and vacuum after a few hours. In addition, check to see if anyone walking in the house has itchy, scaly feet. If so, treat for athlete's foot with a fungicide cream for a few weeks and then reapply baking soda to carpets. If you don't treat the athlete's foot, the carpet odor will return.

Many carpet cleaning products contain potent VOCs, such as naphthalene and perchloroethylene, which are very toxic and potentially carcinogenic to both animals and humans.[25,26,27] Due to increasing public pressure, many companies are now providing carpet and upholstery cleaning services with fewer chemicals. Take the time to do some research and find a reputable carpet-cleaning company. If you have your own carpet shampooer, search for a non-toxic product. Be wary of companies that misleadingly market their toxic products with the "green" or "all- natural" label as happens in other industries. There are some agencies, such as Green Seal (greenseal.org), which has been around since 1989, that provide certification for companies producing truly safer products. By doing a quick search on their website, you will find companies that offer safe, non-toxic products, such as carpet and upholstery cleaners.

Many carpet-cleaning companies will ask if you want the carpet treated with a stain deflector. Scotchgard, a very popular 3M product, has been around for a long time. When applied to fabric, upholstery or carpeting, this material both repels water and prevents staining. In 1999, the EPA started an investigation into Scotchgard because it contained PFOA and PFOS, which, if you remember from the earlier discussion of Teflon, are biopersistent, disease-causing chemicals, now present throughout the world. 3M stopped production of PFOS in 2002 and then reformulated Scotchgard with a different chemical, perfluorobutanesulfonic acid (PFBS), which is less biopersistent than PFOA and PFOS.[28] The half-life of PFBS in humans is a little less than one month.[29] This means it will take your body just under two months to clear out 75% of the amount your skin absorbs from one exposure. So, if you handle clothing treated with Scotchgard, sit on a couch treated with Scotchgard, and/or walk barefoot on carpet treated with Scotchgard once every couple of months, you will begin to bioaccumulate larger and larger concentrations of this particle in your body. I used to apply Scotchgard to my carpets, but I've since stopped. Although it's nice to have stain-free carpets and easy-to-clean upholstery, I've eliminated this product and all products like it from my home.

By modifying habits, the need for stain-free materials can be significantly reduced. Taking off your shoes before entering the house and by either wearing slippers or socks while walking in your home will help keep your carpets clean. If you limit food preparation and dining to the kitchen area or to rooms with hard flooring, there will be fewer stains to worry about. If pets run from outside to inside, either put down hard-surface flooring or deal with the stains by spot cleaning and vacuuming frequently.

Air fresheners

No one wants to have a home that smells bad. The first material used to change a home's odor was incense, which dates back thousands of years. Since the 1940s, however, air freshener technology has become much more sophisticated. Now, air fresheners utilize different chemicals that interface and react with your olfactory system (sense of smell) and employ new efficient techniques for dispersal.

Some deodorizing products, including Febreze, emit VOCs such as 1,4 dichlorobenzene (1,4-DCB), the main ingredient in mothballs and deodorant blocks for restroom toilets and urinals. 1,4-DCB is carcinogenic in mice.[30] Acute exposure to this chemical in humans can cause irritated eyes and skin and a sore throat,[31] while chronic inhalation can affect the liver, skin, and nervous system.[32] Reduced lung function from chronic inhalation has also been reported.[33] Chronic oral ingestion of this chemical is associated with deterioration of the brain, a condition called leukoencephalopathy.[34] Although the EPA considers this chemical to have low toxicity when inhaled, avoiding frequent inhalation is a good idea. When in a public restroom, it may be unavoidable to breathe in this VOC, but you have a choice at home.

In 2007, the Natural Resources Defense Council (NRDC) released a study that tested fourteen air-freshening products on the market. As ironic as it seems, the council's report stated that 86% of these air freshening products released phthalates into the air. As mentioned previously, these endocrine-disrupting chemicals can affect normal hormone production and cause birth defects and reproductive problems. In this study, even brands that touted their products as "all-natural" and "unscented" contained phthalates. Discouragingly, none of these products mentioned phthalates under their ingredient panels.[35]

More preferable are the many natural products available to clean up odors from your home. First of all, if you recognize the source of an odor, try to remove it and/or clean the area with a natural cleanser. As mentioned previously, indoor plants will freshen your air and clear out VOCs. Sodium bicarbonate (baking soda) absorbs odors effectively and safely and can be sprinkled on carpets and placed in closets, bathrooms, and in the refrigerator, where it will remain effective for months. Potpourri and essential oils can add fragrance to the home. Be cautious, though, not to burn paraffin candles or use products containing synthetic fragrances in your home or you will increase the indoor concentration of VOCs.

Furniture care

There are cleaning agents specifically designed for wood, fabric, leather upholstery, metal surfaces, and hard plastics and resins. As with all other cleaning materials, check out the EWG website to see how your preferred products rate. Do some research to see if you can make a simple alternative solution at home to save yourself some money and time and to rid yourself of additional chemicals in your home. Some wood polishers, such as Pledge, contain a long list of chemicals, whereas Murphy's oil soap is a more natural product, containing a vegetable oil base, propylene glycol, synthetic fragrance, and EDTA, a metal chelator. A home recipe for a simple wood polisher can be made by mixing 4 tbsp. of olive oil, 1/2 cup white vinegar, and 1/2 tsp lemon juice. Shake the mixture up in a small bottle and label it. This product will last a long while. Dusting can be achieved with a feather duster or a dusting cloth with minimal chemical infusion. Try a microfiber dust rag. These cloths, as discussed previously, are amazing and will help you clean your furniture surfaces, often without any need for a spray or polish.

Laundry care

Laundry products include detergents, bleaches, fabric softeners, stain pretreatment sticks and solutions, and dryer sheets. These products all contain industry recipes to optimize effectiveness. Check out the EWG website and see if you are content with your chosen cleaning product. If not, see if you can find a detergent or stain remover with a higher rating.

There are naturally occurring surfactants and many products take advantage of natural cleaning solutions. One impressive natural surfactant is produced from a tree indigenous to the Himalayas known as the soap berry tree. The berry shells from this tree contain a surfactant known as saponin. These shells, commonly known as soap nuts, are sold and marketed by many companies. Soap nuts do not produce tons of bubbles or foam and do not clean quite as efficiently or completely as an industrial product in a laundry machine or dishwasher, but they are very useful for gentle cleaning and will certainly work well enough for most cleaning jobs around the house. Soap nut solution can also be sprayed on plants to keep insects away.

In order to extract the saponin from the nut, either boil the nuts in water for 10-20 minutes, or place five or six nuts in a laundry sack and put the sack in with the clothing when doing a load of laundry. When the wash is finished, remove the bag and let it air dry for reuse. A single bag containing half a dozen soap nuts may last for six loads, depending on the type of washer you use, and whether or not you have hard or soft water. If your water is hard, add one or two more nuts to the laundry or 1/2 a cup of baking soda if your clothes are particularly dirty. Laundry softeners and dryer sheets are not needed when cleaning with soap nuts. These nuts reduce static cling and produce softer clothes, naturally. If you choose to try soap nuts, test the solution on a single piece of clothing before washing a whole load.

Laundry is one of the most common uses of household bleach. Try to omit bleach and instead pour either one cup of hydrogen peroxide, one cup of lemon juice, one cup of borax (a form of baking soda), or 1/2 cup of vinegar into your laundry. You can pour any of these solutions directly on stains before running the washing machine. Non-chlorine bleach is a safer choice than chlorine bleach and is referred to as an oxygen bleach as it uses hydrogen peroxide as its active ingredient instead of chlorine.

Fabric softeners and dryer sheets help reduce the static electricity that develops when clothes are spun in a dryer, known as "static cling." Although fabric softeners were initially created to make fabrics softer to the touch, the chemical composition of fabric softeners was later changed to make them "anti-static." Dryer sheets arose in the 1960s to avoid the inconvenience of timing the addition of fabric softener to the washing machine after the first wash cycle. Dryer sheets are small polyester cloths infused with fabric softener and fragrance which can be placed into the dryer with damp clothes. As the dryer spins, the softener and fragrance chemicals coat your clothing. The list of chemicals that make up the fragrance, of course, is proprietary information. These sheets are known to produce VOCs which can cause adverse health effects, including allergies.[36] Dryer balls or even an old sneaker will also reduce static cling. If you like your clothes to smell fresh, you could create a small bag with lavender and throw it in the dryer, or drip a few drops of an essential oil onto the dryer balls or a small clean rag and place it in the dryer with your clothes for five minutes at the end of the drying cycle. Using dryer sheets is an unnecessary source of chemical exposure.

Spiritual cleansing

Many believe that if a house isn't spiritually cleansed in addition to vacuuming, dusting, and surface washing, the house won't be truly clean. Smudging is an ancient ceremonial technique in which sacred plants, such as sage, are burned indoors to cleanse stagnant energy and remove negativity. Many techniques for smudging exist. Typically, the practitioner will ignite a bundle of sage and then blow out the flame, leaving the leaves to smolder and smoke. By using a feather or one's hand, the sacred smoke is then waved to surround and cleanse the body. Next, the smoking organic material is brought through the home or other interior space to be cleansed. Smoke is waved gently to fill each room, including the room's corners and closet. While performing this ritual, an intention is held that the smoke is removing any negative energies that have accumulated within the space. Once the process is over, energy within the room is renewed.

Although articles have deemed this practice as having tangible, biochemical and physiological value, such as disinfecting the air,[37] I find smudging to be most useful as a spiritual treatment. If your home or specific rooms in your home make you feel low in energy, try smudging them with sage and see how you feel afterwards.

Making smart choices

House cleaning is an important way to make the home a safe and healthy environment. By making educated decisions concerning which cleaning products to use in the home, one can limit the ingestion and contact exposure to thousands of chemicals that permeate the household cleaning industry. Be creative and be safe by first doing your own research and then switching to safer, non-toxic alternatives, and/or by making your own cleaning products from common kitchen staples.

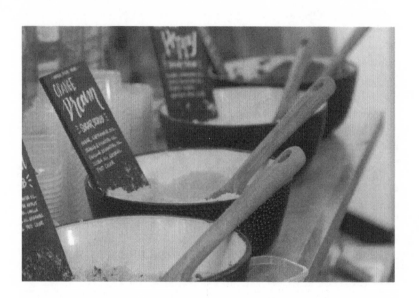

Chapter 7

PERSONAL CARE PRODUCTS

The personal care product industry produces a huge, diverse array of products ranging from hair and skin care products to colognes, deodorants, etc. With few exceptions, such as dental products, most personal care products are designed to cleanse, beautify, or otherwise tend to the skin, hair, and nails.

The skin is considered the largest organ of the body. Although it doesn't look like an organ as a liver or a pancreas does, it has several vital functions. First and foremost, the skin is a protector, providing us with a shield from physical, chemical, and biological entities that could otherwise harm us. The skin also allows our bodies to either expel or conserve water and regulate both our internal temperature and the internal concentration of salts by constricting or dilating tiny blood vessels. Our skin, when exposed to sunlight, helps our body to produce vitamin D, a vitamin critical for a healthy immune system as well as for the production of healthy bones, cartilage, and connective tissue. Nerves in the skin process and transmit information to the brain, providing us with a sense of touch and allowing us to interact physically with the world beyond the senses of sight, smell, and hearing.

Before discussing personal care products, it is important to first understand that the skin isn't just a simple covering over your "insides," but is composed of three layers: the epidermis, dermis, and subcutaneous tissue.

The surface of the epidermis, the outermost layer of the skin, is lined with keratin and dried-up cells. There are many different cell types in the epidermis, including hair, nails, and the sweat glands. The epidermis is a dynamic structure—cells constantly move toward the skin surface, where they die and slough off, and are replaced by new cells. In this way, shallow cuts and scrapes can heal.

Pilo-sebaceous units in the skin produce hair and sweat. Hair protects us from the rain, wind, and sun and also helps to dissipate sebum, our sweat gland product, from the skin surface. All hair follicles have the same structure. The spacing and distribution of hair is determined by one's genetic expression. Because of societal emphasis on one's image, the marketplace is flooded with products that make your hair look "better," which could mean a different color, thicker, softer, straighter, curlier, more manageable, or shinier.

Fingernails provide us with protection. They provide us with an enhanced sense of touch and help us feel and hold on to small objects. Fingernails grow two to three times faster than toenails; the average fingernail grows approximately 3 1/2 mm a month.[1] Covering the nail with polish and other ornaments is a huge industry.

Beneath the epidermis sits the dermis, a layer composed primarily of cells that produce a large protein called collagen. Cells in the dermis are constantly producing and breaking down collagen in order to provide the skin its structure and substance. Collagen allows skin to resist deformation and tearing. Many products have capitalized on the idea that collagen makes your skin younger-looking and more resilient. This is true, but collagen molecules are specifically created and placed within a matrix designed by your dermis. Collagen cannot simply be applied to the skin or be injected into the dermis to be incorporated into this matrix. Injected collagen, a popular dermal filler, becomes reabsorbed quickly by the body.[2] However, the understanding of how this matrix breaks down in older skin and how it can be stimulated to produce new collagen is increasing. More recently, the oral ingestion of supplements, including hydrolyzed collagen, hyaluronic acid, and other amino acids, has been shown to improve skin elasticity.[3]

Beneath the dermis lies a layer of subcutaneous tissue. This layer contains fat cells and gives the skin thickness and separates it from the underlying muscle. Skin thickness varies in different parts of the body. For instance, the skin on the eyelid is much thinner than the skin on the back. The components of the skin differ in each location as well. For example, the skin on the palms of the hand and the soles of the feet normally contain many more nerves than the skin on the back.

The skin surface is home to billions of beneficial bacteria and fungi, which together form the skin microbiome. This forms a protective layer against harmful or pathogenic bacteria and other microorganisms.[4] The normally occurring bacteria on your skin are in balance with each other and with you. Without a healthy skin microbiome, the immune system can suffer and become overwhelmed, resulting in greater susceptibility to infections and allergies.[5] Bacteria comprising the normal microbiome have also been shown to produce antioxidant enzymes that protect skin cells.[6]

The strains of bacteria that comprise your microbiome depend on the moisture content of the skin and whether or not the skin is exposed to the elements.[7] For example, the strains of bacteria that live on the skin under your arms are different from the types of bacteria that live on the back of your hand, because bacteria and yeasts need specific conditions in order to flourish. In areas with persistent moisture and warmth, such as between the toes and legs, and in other areas where skin overlaps skin, some microorganisms, particularly yeasts, can overpopulate, causing a rash, odor and itchiness.

Skin can become damaged and compromised by sources of electromagnetic energy. Different wavelengths of energy, such as infrared, visible light, and UV radiation, can cause skin reactions, ranging from the sensation of warmth to interference with cellular DNA, which can cause skin cancer. UV radiation has been shown to cause large areas of damage to the skin's integrity, making the skin more permeable to toxins.[8]

There are two categories of compounds that can interact with the skin: organic and inorganic. Organic compounds are, with a few exceptions, naturally occurring and synthetic molecules that contain at least one carbon atom. Organic compounds are more easily absorbed through intact skin than inorganic compounds. If an organic compound, such as acetone, contacts your skin, you will quickly feel irritation in your eyes and a strange taste in your mouth, clearly indicating that the chemical has been absorbed through your skin and travelled through the bloodstream. In general, fat-soluble organic compounds pass through the skin more easily than water-soluble compounds.

Inorganic compounds include salts, metals, minerals, water, etc. The skin has a low permeability for most inorganic compounds, meaning that when inorganic compounds interface with intact skin, most will not be absorbed or be able to pass through it. Notable exceptions include several toxic metals, including lead and arsenic. Whereas some heavy metals, such as mercury, cannot penetrate the skin in elemental form, they may do so when bonded to an organic compound, such as methylmercury. In addition, if inorganic compounds are turned into nanoparticles 40 nm in diameter or smaller, they may also penetrate intact skin.[9] Many personal care products and some pharmaceuticals are incorporating nanotechnology to deliver inorganic compounds into the body through intact skin.

Our daily interactions with solvents, organic compounds, and nanoparticles are more common than you might think. Cosmetics, nail polish remover, lotions, deodorants, and skin cleansers have compounds that can damage the microbiome, penetrate the skin, and potentially cause damage to the skin and to the body's internal systems.[10]

Exposure to organic and inorganic compounds is not limited to the skin. Personal care products, such toothpastes, mouthwashes, lipsticks, and other types of "make-up" can be ingested orally. Products used in the genital area can penetrate into the vagina, urethra, and anus. For many years it was debated whether or not talc, an inorganic element used in baby powders and other hygiene products, was causing ovarian cancer. A study published in May 2016 confirmed this association in the scientific literature.[11]

Most personal care products claim to offer qualities such as beauty, youthfulness, appeal, attractiveness, and cleanliness. According to Environmental Working Group research, women, on average, use twelve personal care products each day, whereas men use about six. Personal care products designed for infants and babies include wipes, bubble baths, and baby shampoo. Most everyone in the Western world uses at least a few personal care products each day.

Believe it or not, companies are able to put potentially dangerous ingredients into their personal care products without any labeling requirements. These might consist of compounds that change colors, consistencies, fragrances, or preservatives to prolong shelf life. Although most manufacturers test their products for the potential for localized skin irritation and allergy, they devote few resources to study the potential for long-term systemic health effects, such as the development of cancer or the disturbance of the reproductive and endocrine systems.

The Environmental Working Group found that, on average, women exposed themselves to 168 different chemicals each day and men to 85 through the use of personal care products. These chemicals range from innocuous ingredients such as collagen to potentially carcinogenic compounds, such as formaldehyde, and endocrine-disrupting compounds, such as propylparabens, a common preservative. Heavy metals such as cadmium and lead have been found in some products, including lipstick. In 2007, David Steinman, the publisher and editor of *Healthy Living Magazine*, had an independent lab test different bath products for his children's use and discovered that some of them, including those labeled "natural" and "organic," contained 1,4-dioxane. This potentially carcinogenic chemical forms as a byproduct when the petrochemical ethylene oxide is added to foaming agents, a step in the production of products that make bubbles. A few of the more common compounds used in this industry are listed in Table 8. But keep in mind there is no way for a consumer to know if the products they use contain any of these chemicals because of the lack of labeling requirements.

Table 8. Common chemicals used in the personal care products industry

Parabens	Triclosan
Phthalates	Formaldehyde
Quaternium-15	DEP
DMDM hydantoin	1,4 Dioxane
Lead Acetate	Nanoparticles
DEA, TEA, MEA	BHA, BHT
PVP, VA copolymer	Sodium lauryl/laureth sulfate
Fragrance	Propylene glycol and PEGs
Diazolidinyl urea/midazolidinyl urea	

In 2015, Senators Dianne Feinstein and Susan Collins introduced a bill in the Senate known as the Personal Care Products Safety Act, designed to strengthen the FDA's authority to regulate the chemicals placed in personal care products. The bill would require the FDA to study and evaluate a minimum of five ingredients per year to determine their safety and affirm their appropriate use. The first five ingredients to be studied would be:

1. Diazolidinyl urea: a preservative used in a wide range of products, including deodorants, shampoos, conditioners, bubble baths, and skin lotions.
2. Lead acetate: a color additive used to formulate hair dyes.
3. Methylene glycol/formaldehyde: chemicals used in hair treatments.
4. Propyl paraben: a preservative used in shampoos, conditioners, and skin lotions.
5. Quaternium-15: a preservative used in shampoos, creams, and cleansers.

The Personal Care Products Safety Act is a step in the right direction, but as of the time of this writing, in July 2017, it has yet to be passed.

There are hundreds, if not thousands, of different naturally occurring and synthetically produced chemical compounds currently in use. In addition, new compounds are being developed by chemists every year. The good news is that there is growing attention to this problem in the media and new healthier alternatives are surfacing all of the time. Even big box stores, such as Walmart and Sam's Club, are requiring suppliers to submit their products for ingredient analysis and review before they are sold.

With free trade agreements, the American consumer needs to be concerned with not only what American industries are putting into their products, but also what other countries are adding. There are several agencies in place, such as the Personal Care Products Council International Committee and NSF International, that try to regulate the industry, but it's a big world out there and there are tens of thousands of ingredients and chemicals used in the creation of millions of products.

What can you do today?

First, protect your children by limiting the number of products they use and evaluating those products carefully. Because of their smaller size, the effect of chemicals absorbed through their skin can be more damaging than in an adult. Girls exposed to estrogen, endocrine-disrupting chemicals, or placental elements in hair care products may go through puberty too early.[12] An earlier onset of menarche[13] and the use of personal care products containing estrogens[14] are both associated with an increased risk of future breast cancer. Research and educate yourself the best you can.

Until the industry is more tightly regulated, there are two ways you can reduce your exposure to the toxic chemicals in personal care products. The first is to limit what you use. A great first step would be to become more conscious of what products you use daily. Make a list and see if there are any products you can do without.

The safety of a given product has as much to do with how and where it is applied as it does with its ingredients. Be most critical about products that are applied to large areas of the body for the longest amount of time. Soaking in a tub filled with bath gels or bubble bath will provide potentially harmful chemicals a larger surface area to contact and a longer exposure than a shampoo quickly lathered and rinsed off. Lotions, creams, and powders that are applied to large areas of skin should be chosen carefully.

Products that are applied to smaller skin surface areas, but are potentially more toxic, include hair dyes, nail polish, fragrances, deodorant, and even baby wipes. Other products applied to smaller parts of the body are generally less concerning, including eye shadow, blush, hand soap, nail polish, and nail polish remover.

Heavy metal toxicity may be an exception, however. The FDA did an investigation into the lipstick market in 2012 and found low levels of lead contamination in every sample tested, with lead levels measuring up to 7.19 parts per million (ppm).[15] This created a stir in the industry. Further testing showed that heavy metals, including lead and cadmium, can be found in trace amounts in many different cosmetics, such as lipstick, skin creams, foundation, mascara, blush, eyeliner, and others.[16] As these metals are impurities, they are not required to be listed on the label.[17] The FDA has set a maximum contaminant level of lead in cosmetics at 10 ppm. Lipsticks are therefore considered safe if used correctly, but what is the correct use of lipstick? Is it proper use to eat or drink liquids while wearing lipstick? If one wears lipstick, should they refrain from licking their lips or kissing another on the lips? It has been proven that a slow, chronic intake of small quantities of lead or cadmium over time can lead to bioaccumulation and be toxic and damaging to many organ systems, including the heart, kidneys, bones, and liver.[18]

Many are on the search for safer personal care products. Before shopping for "organic" personal care products though, understand that the FDA has no definition for the terms "organic" or "natural" in the personal care product industry and thus no regulations exist. A company can print either or both of those words on a product label, regardless of the undisclosed list of ingredients. Claiming a synthetic personal care product to be organic can be a deceptive marketing technique.

Consumer advocacy groups have formed to help those concerned better know what they are buying. One group, the Natural Products Association, provides a "natural seal" on products whose ingredients come from renewable sources found in nature that have no suspected human health risk. An excellent online resource available to the public is the Good Guide, at www.GoodGuide.com. This website rates and reviews personal care products, food items, and products used in the home for their safety. The Environmental Working Group regularly updates a wonderful online resource at www.EWG.org/SkinDeep that provides information on a large number of commercially available cosmetics for sale in the US. This website also provides a mobile app for ready access while shopping. Another convenient online resource is the mobile app "Think Dirty." This app ranks the safety of specific products in the marketplace on a scale of 1 to 10 and offers cleaner alternatives.

If you have favorite products that are not evaluated by any of these resources, a few observations may give you a hint as to a product's contents. For example, if a personal care product is formulated without a preservative, it will most likely be packaged in a smaller container and will have a limited shelf life with an expiration date. If a product requires you to shake before use, that is an indication that fewer chemicals have been added as compared to a homogeneous colloidal suspension without the need for shaking. Petroleum-based fragrance products such as colognes and perfumes are composites of many different synthetic chemicals blended together. Fragrance chemicals are exempt from the list of required ingredients to be included on a label in the personal care product industry due to a loophole in the Fair Packaging and Labeling Act of 1973. There is no regulation behind the words "fragrance free" or "unscented." If these words are used, the product may contain masking fragrances which can cause hypersensitivity reactions in people who are allergic to fragrances.[19]

Sunblock and suntan lotion

The sun-protection industry boomed following the invention of the SPF system in 1962. There are sunblocks for children, sunblocks that moisturize, water-resistant sunblocks, sunblocks for sensitive skin, and sunblocks that include an insect repellent.[20] In December 2012, the FDA enforced labeling requirements for manufacturers to accurately disclose the ingredients and effectiveness of each product. Terms such as "waterproof" or "sweat-proof," are no longer allowed because they are misleading. If a product is labeled "water resistant," it must specify how long the product will typically stay on the skin while the wearer is in water. Warning labels are now placed on tanning agents containing values of SPF 2-14 stating that the product has not been shown to help prevent skin cancer or early skin aging.[21]

As a consumer, it is important to understand what the SPF system means. The SPF determination is based on a specific application thickness and frequency of use. If properly applied, a product with an SPF of 2 would allow one to stay out in the sun twice as long as if not wearing any product. A product with an SPF 4 rating would allow one to stay in the sun 4 times longer, etc. The new labeling requirements allow an SPF range from 2 through 50+, with products with an SPF over 50 designated as 50+.

The band of wavelengths that make up the UV radiation spectrum is subdivided into UV-A, UV-B, and UV-C. The standard SPF rating indicates the degree to which the sunblock protects the skin from UV-B radiation only. Sunblocks that protect from UV-B radiation only will help protect the skin from sunburn and from the potential of squamous cell cancer, a less severe form of skin cancer.[22] UV-A radiation, however, is associated with the development of melanoma, the most dangerous type of skin cancer. UV-A measurement standards are currently being developed. Sunblocks that protect from both UV-B and UV-A radiation, if used properly, are referred to as broad-spectrum sunscreens. "If used properly" usually means that you need to put the sunscreen product on thirty minutes before going out in the sun and reapply at least every two hours during exposure, regardless of whether or not you go swimming or are actively sweating. Broad spectrum sunscreen products are becoming increasingly available, but there is no research indicating that their frequent application prevents melanoma and basal cell carcinoma. A big risk factor for developing future skin cancer, including melanoma, is a history of frequent sunburns, at any age.[23] So take precautions to not get burned.

Sunblocks use many different chemicals that are unique to each product and manufacturer. According to the Environmental Working Group's Sunscreen Guide for 2017,

65% of the non-mineral sunscreen products tested were found to contain oxybenzone, an endocrine disruptor shown to have weak estrogen and strong anti-androgenic effects.[24] I would suggest finding a sunscreen that does not contain this chemical ingredient.

Choosing a sunblock is an important decision, as you'll be applying large swaths of product to your skin every day, and perhaps several times a day. Do some research and purchase a broad-spectrum sunblock with as high a health safety rating as you can find in a product with a minimum SPF of 15. If you are planning to spend a long time in the sun, use the sunblock properly, and in addition, wear sunglasses, a hat, and, if available, spend at least some of the day sitting under a tree or umbrella. Some sunshine is good for you, but too much, whether or not you are wearing sunblock, can cause skin cancer.

Soaps and cleansers

When choosing a soap, consider that plain soap and water are all one needs to clean unwanted bacteria and viruses off the skin. Antibacterial soaps and other antibacterial skin products are toxic to the microbiome. The active ingredient in most of these products is triclosan, a known endocrine disruptor. Antibacterial soaps were everywhere in years past, but in 2016, the FDA ordered manufacturers to remove the antibacterial label from consumer soaps.

Many personal care products can be made at home. Many websites and books teach how to create organic formulations from household ingredients. The simplest personal care product one can formulate at home is a skin moisturizer/body oil. Just open up a jar of coconut oil and apply! Coconut oil is a healthy cooking oil and is also a wonderful way to keep your skin looking youthful and healthy.

Two additional personal care products that can easily be made are toothpaste and body scrubs. Consumer toothpastes typically contain everything from nanoparticles and triclosan to sodium laureth sulfate and fluoride. Artificial sweeteners may also be added, particularly to children's toothpaste. It's easy to avoid these toxins, and particularly important to do so if you have gingivitis or gums that bleed when brushed.

A brush and a mildly abrasive material are all that you need to take off the daily film that develops on teeth. Commonly used abrasive materials include baking soda, sea salt, or bentonite clay. By mixing the abrasive with some water to form a paste and then adding a drop of essential oil, such as cinnamon or peppermint, you will have a palatable toothpaste. If you prefer your toothpaste with a creamy consistency, mix the abrasive with a bit of coconut oil. The quantity of each ingredient is a personal choice.

A body scrub is a simple bath product to make. Commercial varieties are usually filled with synthetic fragrances, dyes, and additives to increase shelf life. The two most common ingredients used to scrub the body are sugar and salt, both crystalline at room temperature. By rubbing the crystals on the skin, dead skin cells are effectively scraped off, a process called exfoliation. The result is a layer of shinier, healthier-looking skin. Many prefer salt because it relaxes muscles, can act as an antiseptic, and will provide a more intense exfoliation. Sugar is not quite as abrasive as salt and many prefer sugar scrubs for more sensitive, softer areas of the body. Regardless of which you choose, the process for creating a scrub is the same. In order to have the crystals available in a spreadable medium, it is necessary to put these crystals in an oil so they don't dissolve. Any liquid oil of your choice will do. Some prefer infused oils, while others may choose almond oil or olive oil. In any case, fill a small jar with the salt or sugar and then cover it with oil, and you have your own scrub. It's really that simple. To make the concoction fragrant, add aroma from an essential oil or throw in dried flowers or leaves of your favorite herb. Feel free to experiment. For a gentle exfoliant, try oatmeal instead of sugar or salt. If you have been a commercial consumer for body scrubs, you'll most likely wonder why you've spent so much money on these "luxurious" products after you see how easy they are to make at home.

In conclusion

These are just a few suggestions on how to get started making your own personal care products. I'd suggest making one product now, see how it goes, and if you are happy with the result, try to make a second. If you have an adventurous spirit, you can try to make most everything you use, including deodorant. You'll be surprised at how good you ultimately feel, not only because of your own ingenuity but also from the decreased load of daily toxins.

PART III
ENERGY AND SPIRIT

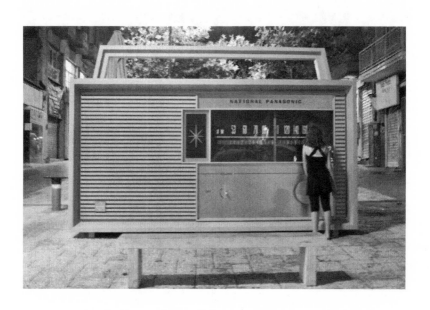

Chapter 8
SOUND

Sound and music can have a profound fortifying or enervating effect on one's well-being. Noise is a noxious form of pollution that can have both psychological and physiological effects.

What is sound?

Sound is technically a sensual stimulus, meaning that it is something we can perceive with a sense organ, the ear. Sound is the result of the transmission of mechanical vibrations generated at a source by the compression and rarefaction of matter. Sound cannot exist in an instant, for it takes time for the wave to travel a given distance. The speed of sound is dependent on the matter that the sound is traveling through. Sound travels almost a million times slower than light through air, at approximately 770 miles per hour, depending on the speed and direction of wind, temperature, air pressure, and humidity. Sound travels approximately four times faster in water than it does in air.

All matter is in a state of constant vibration. Since all matter vibrates, all matter creates sound, even though we may not be able to hear it. A sound's character is determined by the rapidity of the vibration, referred to as the oscillation frequency. Faster vibrations will generate higher-frequency sounds while slower vibrations will generate lower sounds. Sounds heard by the human ear are between the frequencies of 20 and 20,000 Hz (cycles per second).

A repetitive oscillation frequency will produce a melodic tone. For example, the tone produced by a periodic wave with an oscillating frequency at 440 cycles per second will generate a sound corresponding to the musical note "A."

When an oscillating frequency is variable and not repetitive, the sound will be percussive or atonal, like a drum beat.

Most music comes from the layering of multiple periodic frequencies, which creates synchronous tones in succession. To give the music structure and rhythm, non-periodic percussive beats are added, creating a complex overlay of many different types of vibration and frequency. Some of these frequencies are louder than others (referred to as dynamics), which adds further complexity and depth of the music.

Volume is determined by the amplitude of the sound wave. The larger the amplitude, the more energy the tone carries, and the louder the sound will be to our ears. Loudness is quantified in units on the decibel (dB) scale, a logarithmic scale. Because the scale is logarithmic, each increase of 10 dB represents a 10-fold increase in the energy of the sound. The dB levels for several typical household sounds are listed in Table 9.

Table 9. Common household noises with corresponding dB levels

Watch ticking - 20 dB
Conversation - 40 dB
Dishwasher, microwave - 60 dB
Garbage disposal, vacuum cleaner - 80 dB
Lawnmower - 90 dB
Hairdryer - 100 dB

A hairdryer is therefore 100 times louder than a typical garbage disposal. Sound dissipates over distance following the "inverse square law." So, a dishwasher might have a 60-dB noise level if you measure the sound level five feet from the dishwasher itself, but if you walk ten feet away, thereby doubling your distance from the appliance, the sound intensity would drop by four times.

Mechanism of hearing

The ear is a sensitive instrument that gathers and, in a sense, decodes sound into electrochemical impulses. The brain then has the job of interpreting and reacting to the sound. The hearing mechanism, referred to as the auditory system, is composed of three distinct units: the external auditory canal, the middle ear, and the inner ear.

The outermost segment of the ear, a short channel known as the external auditory canal, ends at the eardrum, known as the tympanum or tympanic membrane. Sound gathered by the outer folds of the ear travels into the auditory canal and bounces off the tympanum, causing it to vibrate. Sound waves are thus transmuted into mechanical vibrations of the eardrum, which then transmit the sound information into the middle ear.

The middle ear is an air-filled chamber that houses three tiny bones, known as ossicles, which form a bridge from the tympanic membrane to another thin membrane called the oval window, the entrance to the inner ear. Because of their size, orientation, and position, the ossicles are able to accurately deliver a minified representation of the vibrations from one membrane to the other.

Once the sound vibrations are transmitted to the oval window, they have reached the inner ear. In the inner ear is the cochlea, a coiled structure that looks like a snail shell from the outside. The cochlea is filled with fluid and projecting from its floor are tiny hairs known as cilia. The cilia are at a standstill in complete silence, but if a vibration hits the oval window, the fluid in the cochlea will vibrate, causing the tiny cilia to move back and forth. The movement of these cilia causes an electrochemical impulse that is transmitted to the brain through the auditory nerve, where it is interpreted as sound. Louder sounds excite more cilia.

The auditory system and, in particular, the cochlea, are much more complex than what I just described. But this brief overview will give you an understanding that we are able to hear because of an intricate multi- chamber system that translates sound waves into mechanical vibrations and then into electrochemical impulses. The ability to hear ultimately depends on the movement of cilia in the cochlea and the transmission of impulses from the cochlea, up the auditory nerves, and into the brain.

The ears never turn off. Studies have shown that the auditory system begins to function before birth, at around six months of gestation.[1] So the fetus hears during the second half of pregnancy. From this point forward, the ears are always "on," even during sleep, while in a comatose state, or under anesthesia.[2] Hearing is said to be the last sense to go. The brain analyzes every sound that causes the eardrum to vibrate. If the brain recognizes a pattern in the sound, the importance of the sound will diminish as we become more passively aware of the sound. If, however, the sound is unrecognizable or doesn't conform to a recognizable pattern, the brain will actively listen and try to understand and figure out what it is hearing. Unrecognizable sounds can and will distract you from activities requiring mental focus.[3]

The hearing mechanism is interconnected with other systems in the body. In fact, many of the cranial nerves that exit the brain stem are affected in some way or another by the auditory system. The 10th cranial nerve, known as the vagus nerve, has attachments to the tympanic membrane. After leaving the head, the vagus nerve innervates organs in the neck, chest, abdomen, and pelvis. This means that the signals traveling between the brain and the body's organs also contain vibratory information from the eardrums. Sound can have a near-direct effect on the whole body and does not have to be interpreted by the brain in order to cause a systemic reflexive response.[4] Think about the immediate systemic effects that occur when one hears a baby cry.

Resonance and harmonics

The auditory system is not the only pathway by which sound can affect the body. Sounds can transfer energy directly to the body, bypassing the ears through resonance. Resonance is the ability for energy to transfer from one structure to another through a matching of frequencies. A common example of this is the case of the empty crystal wine glass and the opera singer. The opera singer can ping the side of the glass to listen to the tone made by the empty glass. That pitch represents the resonant frequency of the glass and therefore the frequency at which the glass will absorb and transmit energy. If the opera singer sings the resonant frequency or "note" of the glass precisely, at a sufficient loudness and duration, the glass will absorb the sound energy from the voice. This energy can cause the glass to vibrate and eventually shatter if it is strong enough. A less dramatic example might be to place two acoustic instruments, such as guitars, next to each other. If you play one of the open strings on one guitar, the same string on the other guitar will vibrate and produce sound because the sound energy produced by the first guitar will be absorbed by the second guitar's string. What is really interesting about this phenomenon, though, is that most acoustic sounds, and our voices in particular, will resonate with more than one frequency through harmonics. Harmonics provide the complex layering of sound.

Every cell in the body vibrates, each producing its own frequency. Like cells produce similar frequencies and resonate with each other. Each of the organs in your body and your body as a whole are able to operate as functional units because of resonance. In addition, through harmonics and resonance, we are connected to the world around us. Because of the physics of harmonics, any note played will resonate with anything in the room that is tuned to the same frequency, from a wine glass to structures within the body. Resonance will affect tiny structures with the same tonal value, even if they're beyond our hearing range.

The production of harmonics is much richer with acoustic instruments and the human voice than with electronic music. Depending on the sound source, there may be layers of overtones that are more subtle than the dominant tone and therefore are not clearly discriminated. These overtones, though, are heard by your ears and give the sound a richer, fuller sound, referred to as timbre. These overtones also resonate and transfer energy. Digital sounds will produce fewer harmonics and less resonance. There is a very real experiential difference in hearing a musician play a violin live compared with hearing one played through electronic media.

Unfortunately, most music heard today is through digital media and therefore much of the richness of the music is lost. The notes that you hear are the same, of course, but the harmonics are diminished. Unfortunately, poorer-quality sound has become the norm as many listen to digital music through streaming music apps, MP3 files, and other technologies that utilize data compression software.

Music and sound do not need to be loud to cause resonance. The frequency of the tones, or pitch, is what creates resonance, not the loudness. Think of the body as being composed of billions of tiny wine glasses, each with its own harmonic resonance. The frequency that causes the femur (the long bone in your leg) to absorb energy would be different from the frequency in a strand of DNA. Yet both will demonstrate harmonic resonance and will absorb the energies produced by ambient tones, especially music.

Many spiritual practices, including most religions, include sounds with their prayers. Solitary sounds and monosyllabic words are used in prayer in many religions with Sanskrit origins. These religions subscribe to the idea that the body is divided into seven energy centers called chakras, each connecting to a different level of consciousness. Each chakra has been ascribed a tonal frequency, and gongs and singing bowls tuned to these frequencies can be played to energize each chakra. There are sound healers in practice throughout the world who provide sound treatments to balance and energize the body, mind, and spirit through chakra work.

A single tone produced by a musical instrument or perhaps a singing bowl will transfer energy through harmonic resonance. Add multiple sounds in succession and we have what we call music. The structure of organized sound in music allows our brain to create associations, memories, and even different emotional states based on those memories.[5]

Entrainment

While the tones of music resonate, rhythm produces a phenomenon called entrainment. Have you ever gone into a store that sells cuckoo clocks? If so, you must have noticed that all of the clocks on the wall had pendulums swinging in unison. This synchronization happens automatically and is called entrainment. Entrainment is not limited to cuckoo clocks, but can occur between any two vibrating or oscillating bodies.[6] The human body vibrates and entrains to both internal and external rhythms all the time. People in close proximity to one another for long periods of time can entrain to each other.[7] Mothers and daughters and women who are close friends or roommates with other women will often sync menstrual cycles.[8] Heart rate and breathing rate can synchronize between close individuals or when two people are in face-to-face communication.[9] We are not islands unto ourselves. All things communicate through entrainment with each other.

Entrainment is not a voluntary or conscious decision, but a physical phenomenon. A person's breath, pulse, and brain activity can be modified by entrainment to musical rhythm.[10] This is one of the reasons why singing a lullaby to an agitated infant will calm the baby down.[11] Put on an upbeat, fast song and you will feel energized. Put on a slow song and your pulse will slow and you may become more lethargic.

In order for entrainment to occur, both structures must be physically able to achieve the same vibratory frequency. The closer an object is to a source of oscillation, the more readily it will become entrained. So, if you have two cuckoo clocks on the wall next to each other, they will become more easily entrained than if you had one in an upstairs room and the other in the basement.

Within the human body, entrainment occurs between internal systems all the time. There are many rhythms within the human body, such as the heartbeat, breathing rate, brain wave cycles, circadian rhythms, hormonal cycles, and even molecular rhythms. These are all independent systems from each other, yet they show interdependency through entrainment.[12] For example, if you focus on slowing and controlling your breath during meditation, you will then find your pulse slows down and your brain wave activity slows, both through the process of entrainment.[13]

Classical music and instrumental forms of jazz, blues, and rock all have the ability to cause significant physiological effects through both harmonic resonance and entrainment. A French physician and pioneer in the study of music's physiological effects, Alfred Tomatis, MD, described the ability of classical music, in particular Mozart, to increase intelligence and creativity, reduce stress, and help heal.[14] It has been suggested that listening to the complex patterns of classical music facilitates neuronal growth and results in the development of complex neural networks as the brain "figures out" patterns within the music it is listening to and interpreting.[15] These neural networks can then provide an excellent foundation for the understanding of abstract thought later in life, such as with mathematics and language.[16] Dr. Tomatis called this "The Mozart Effect." Mozart's music is not unique in its ability to stimulate brain development and create these physiological effects,[17] but is a good example of the power that one composer's music can have on the listener's brain development and health.

Add words and a human voice and the music transforms into a powerful vehicle to transmit consciousness and profoundly affect another's state of mind and overall health. Words can bring the listener images that generate thoughts and emotion, referred to as guided imagery. The overall tone of the song, the phrasing of the words, and the dynamics of the piece can all create emotional effects that bring on physiological changes and perhaps create life experiences through manifestation. Many have lived out the same experience as the one described in a song they listened to over and over again. Some would dismiss this as coincidence, but others consider it progressive manifestation. In other words, the listener re-manifests the intention of the artist who originally wrote the song.

From Gregorian chants, tribal songs, and religious prayers, to pop and rap, musical expression has forever shaped society. Music has united groups of people and also caused the splintering of masses who resonate with different artists or styles of music. Music has caused some societies to shift direction. For example, the energy and excitement generated by Elvis Presley caused a profound shift in the consciousness of the youth around the world. Following Elvis, the Beatles did, too. These shifts occurred through and because of their music.

Toxicity

From 2001-2008, one out of eight American kids between the ages of six and nineteen suffered from hearing loss.[18] That number is likely higher today. Overuse of portable music devices with earbuds has contributed to the increasing number of adolescents and adults with noise-induced hearing loss (NIHL).[19] Chronic, excessive loud noise is the second-most common cause for hearing loss in the US, behind aging.[20]

Whereas the impulse noise from an explosion can cause direct trauma to the ear by blowing out the eardrum and damaging the ossicles in the middle ear,[21] it is much more common for NIHL to take dozens of years to develop, as the result from ischemia (decreased blood supply) to the cochlea.[22] Loud sounds cause constriction of blood vessels supplying the cochlea, damaging the cilia inside. In humans, cilia do not have the ability to regenerate, and so once they are damaged, they are gone forever. Continued exposure to loud noise will result in the loss of more and more cilia over time.

NIHL is progressive and dependent on both the loudness of the noise one is exposed to and the number of exposures. "Going deaf" is not usually an instantaneous all-or-none phenomenon. NIHL usually begins in the late twenties or early thirties and can initially manifest as the inability to discriminate between different sounds and/or hypersensitivity to noise. Tinnitus, or ringing in the ears, can also be a sequela to NIHL.

Damage to the cochlea can be even more extensive if you listen to loud music or noise during exercise, when blood flow is diverted to exercising muscles. People who wear earbuds while listening to loud music during a workout are doubling their risk of hearing loss because ischemia to the cochlea is compounded by the additive effects of loud music and exercise.[23] As a general rule of thumb, it is unwise to raise the volume of a device above two-thirds the maximum. If you are trying to have a conversation with your child and they are in the same room with you with earbuds in, and they can't hear you, the volume is too high.

The maximum sound intensity that will not produce hearing loss under normal health conditions, regardless of duration, is 80 dB,[24] about the noise level generated by a garbage disposal or vacuum cleaner. If you are taking medications, know that large doses of aspirin, Tylenol, anti-inflammatories, Lasix, and some antibiotics can lower the threshold for hearing damage.[25,26] When on these medications, take extra precautions to lower your exposure to loud music and other sounds. If you are exposed to loud noise for a prolonged period of time, such as when using a blow dryer, it is best to then take some quiet time afterward to let your ears rest. Let your ears rest for at least fifteen minutes after each hour of exposure to loud noise or music.

Noise can trigger a stress response which results in transient suppression of the immune system.[27] Because of this, bothersome noise, regardless of loudness, should be considered an environmental pollutant. Subtle sounds, such as the whining of a computer monitor or TV screen, the low vibration caused by an old refrigerator, or the creaking of a door, can cause a low level of anxiety.

The home is a place where we want control over our environment. Penetration of noise into the home can be perceived as an inescapable personal violation. Outdoor noises, such as the rumble of trucks rolling down a nearby highway or the roar of planes flying overhead, can be sources of noise pollution in the home which cause a significant amount of stress. Women who live near airports during pregnancy give birth to smaller babies than those who don't.[28] High-pitched sounds, such as those from sirens and alarms, will cause an even greater stress response. If noise is frequent, the resulting chronic stress response can be damaging to the body. Chronic exposure to excessive noise in the home can make one irritable and cause high blood pressure. In children, increased noise in the home has been associated with poorer school performance and decreased learning aptitude.[29]

Even though your mind may be used to noises in the home (through a process called habituation), the body never gets used to them. Chronic irritating noises in the home, particularly during sleep, may cause occupants to develop subconscious anxiety, edginess, or fatigue that won't resolve until the source of noise is removed.[30] Low-frequency sounds with their associated physical vibrations and white noise can be perceived as being particularly irritating.[31] For this reason, I would stay away from white noise players.

Remediation

What can you do to rid the home of unwanted and potentially damaging noise? First, become aware of the sounds in your home and make a list, dividing up the sources of noise into four categories: noises that are part of the everyday functioning of the house, noise that occurs only during a product's use, noise from other people, and noise that enters the house from outside.

Noise from home appliances, such as the HVAC system or furnace, can only be lessened by reducing or stopping their transmission. Concrete walls with air gaps will help eliminate sound transmission, but if you can't rebuild your home, blocking materials such as insulation can also help.

General maintenance around the house will relieve sporadic noises. Lubricant can prevent squeaky doors. Creaking floor planks should be replaced. Dripping faucets and leaky toilets should be fixed. If the laundry machine is on a main floor or upper floor of the home and causes excessive vibration, try and relocate it to the basement to minimize the vibration. If there are rooms in the home that are "noisy" because of echoes and sound reverberation, use carpets, upholstered furniture, and wall hangings or even acoustical ceiling tiles to decrease echo and reverberations.

Noisy housemates may need "sonic boundaries" so everyone in the home has a greater sense of peace and a less stressful environment. Put limits on how loud the TV and other devices can be. Being surrounded by television noise can cause underlying stress. Being surrounded by music one doesn't like may or may not cause a stress response, but will cause entrainment.[32]

Noise infiltrating into your home from the outside is more than likely coming through the windows. Some windows are more soundproof than others. There is a classification system to rate the effectiveness of a window's sound-proofing efficacy, known as the Sound Transmission Class (STC) rating. The STC rating is a logarithmic scale. Single-pane windows typically have an STC in the range of 26 to 28. Dual-pane glass will usually range from 26 to 32 and soundproof windows range from 48 to 54. In general, the thicker the pane of glass, the more sound it will keep out. Double-pane glass will keep out more noise than single-pane glass, as long as there is an air gap between the panes of glass and as long as the glass sheets are not too thin. Glass thickness for a double-pane window should be at least 1/8" for each sheet, preferably thicker. Storm windows that provide a gap of at least 2" between the sets of glass will reduce the transmission of sound even more than double-pane glass. There are many different options to choose from and it is best to contact a window specialist for advice. Make sure that the specialist addresses the STC rating. The windows might be expensive, but you will be much happier in your home after installation.

If sound comes into the home from a common wall, soundproofing and insulation will help, but won't be able to completely block out the noise because sound can transmit around walls, through joists, and through ceilings, referred to as flanking noise. It is best to get an expert opinion from a specialist such as an acoustical engineer before investing to remedy this problem.

If it is impossible to clear your home of unwanted noise, particularly while you are asleep, invest in ear plugs. They are inexpensive and effective. The health benefits to a good night's sleep cannot be overstated. Ear plugs can be made of foam, silicone, or wax, and typically reduce noise levels by 20 to 30 dB. Earplugs don't block out all sound, but enough to create a sense of increased security and relaxation. You will still hear the alarm clock and children knocking on your door in the middle of the night. Placing cotton in the ear is ineffective.

Ear plugs or over-the-ear noise-cancelling headphones are definitely recommended while using noisy equipment in or around your house, such as a table saw, wood chipper, or other noisy power tool. Protect your ears during these tasks.

Sound and music healing

Many healers believe that different tones can be used to heal diseased parts of the body by restoring their normal vibratory frequency through harmonic resonance. Harmonic resonance then leads to emotional clarity and mindful focus. Basic tones generated by Tibetan singing bowls can be used to create an arrangement of harmonics for healing. These bowls are either metallic or made of a quartz crystal. The bowl is played by either striking the rim or rubbing the rim of the bowl with a striker to produce a rich, vibrant tone filled with harmonics. The metallic bowls seem to emit more overtones than the quartz bowls. Some believe that by singing to the bowl and recreating the frequency with your own voice, the harmonic frequencies will be brought within the body and will create a profound state of relaxation akin to yoga, *qi gong*, and other meditation techniques. Simpler sounds create a greater relaxation response. The transference of energy from the bowl to one's body can cause moods and emotions to shift. In a sense, sound can be considered a nutrient for the nervous system.[33]

Music healing differs from sound healing in that music can affect one's emotions and thought through tonal recognition and related associations. Musical tastes vary tremendously. The associations and significance of songs are unique for each person. Even within an individual, the effect of music can be different depending on one's mood and state of focus. What resonates well one day may not do so the next day.

In conclusion

In summary, remove as many noises from your home as you can, and in their place, add tonal sounds and music. Talk radio and talk shows on TV do not cause relaxation, especially these days with shock jocks, screamers, and yellers trying to be heard. If given a choice between talk radio and music, I would suggest listening to music and singing along with the songs you know. If you know how to play an instrument, bring it out and play it a few times a week. If you can sing along with it, all the better. Encourage your children to sing. It's very healthy for everyone to sing.

Tones, rhythm, and lyrics can each have a profound effect on one through resonance, entrainment, and consciousness. With that being said, listen to the music you like to hear when you want to hear it. Hearing depressing songs written by sad people would more easily entrain a person who is feeling sad, but not one is feeling happy and energetic. Listen to upbeat music when you want to be active and filled with energy rather than music that will slow you down. Conversely, if you are trying to relax or prepare for sleep, listen to slow-paced music, for it will slow your heart rate and brain activity, and prompt a restful state.

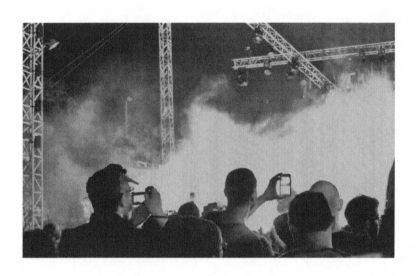

Chapter 9
ELECTROMAGNETIC FIELDS

The electromagnetic spectrum is intricately involved in many aspects of our lives. Frequencies corresponding to the visible light spectrum enable us to see, while those in the infrared range produce heat. Higher frequencies, such as X-rays and gamma rays, have given us diagnostic medical tools, whereas lower-frequency radio waves and microwaves have enabled wireless communication.

As wireless technology continues to expand and becomes implemented into more and more gadgets, there may be unintended consequences from this technology on the electrochemical mechanisms that control our physiology. Electromagnetic radiation (EMR) generated by the use of wireless devices, electrical wiring, and appliances is an effusive and potentially toxic form of energy within and around the home. It is important to understand how EMR is generated and what you can do in your home to lessen unwanted exposure to yourself and your family.

What is electromagnetic frequency (EMF)?

The movement of electrons or any other current through a wire or device will generate both an electric field and a magnetic field, referred to collectively as EMF. The strength of the electric field component increases as the force used to push the electrons through the wire, referred to as the voltage of a system, strengthens. The electric field is always present whether or not a device is operating or turned off. The magnetic field differs from the electric field in that it is only generated by the movement of electrons (current) transmitted through a wire or device over a unit of time. As the current increases, the magnetic field strength increases. When a device is turned off, current ceases and the magnetic field dissipates.

EMR generated by electrical current can be subdivided into extremely low-frequency EMF (ELF-EMF), with frequencies between 1 Hz and 300 kHz, radio frequency (RF), spanning from 300 kHz to 3 GHz, and microwave (MW), with frequencies above 3 GHz.

EMF is a natural phenomenon. In fact, all living beings generate their own electromagnetic fields. The nervous system creates EMF during the transmission of nerve impulses along nerve fibers and within the brain. The earth produces a global magnetic field, a ubiquitous source of EMF. All living beings from bacteria to mammals navigate within the earth's magnetic field, all of the time.[1] The ability to detect the earth's magnetic field allows animals and birds to migrate and navigate in light and in darkness.

The earth's magnetic field has significantly decreased in strength over the past four thousand years. Some believe that a condition in people exists called magnetic deficiency syndrome,[2] in which the earth's magnetic field is not strong enough to provide proper functioning. This condition appears to be improved by the use of magnetic support products. These products produce a static magnetic field, which is a very different type of EMF than those that have been implicated as sources of toxicity.

Manmade sources of EMF are becoming more ubiquitous and are creating localized environmental magnetic anomalies. For animals that fly or swim and travel distances quickly, local magnetic anomalies probably have little effect on their geolocation ability. Animals that move slowly or are relatively stagnant, however, may be affected to a much greater degree by these local phenomena.[3,4] We are surrounded daily by sources of human-made EMF, including power lines, cell phone towers, electrical indoor wiring, electrical appliances, and wireless devices that produce and receive ELF-EMF and RF.

Electric fields can be shielded by walls or other objects, but magnetic fields pass through most material, including drywall, concrete, and more importantly, our skin and soft tissue. As a result, extensive research has been conducted over the last thirty-plus years to assess the potential risks of ELF-EMF and RF to the human population. Many studies have been done in vitro (i.e. bench research in a lab), while other studies are epidemiological, studying disease patterns and symptoms in groups of people in various populations and living conditions. Other researchers have amassed and reviewed groups of individual studies to try and define non-biased trends in larger populations.

Numerous cellular research studies have attempted to define the effects of EMF on specific proteins and receptors in various types of cells, including animal, bacterial, and fungal cells. Researchers have determined that there are proteins in the cell membrane that are activated by specific energies of the electromagnetic spectrum. When activated, they perform their biological actions. We have also discovered that ion gates in cell membranes open up in response to low frequencies.[5] EMF has also been observed to cause vibration and transient deformity of cell membranes, generating heat.[6] Because enzymes are designed to operate within specific temperature ranges, localized increases in temperature can alter enzymatic activity within the affected cell. Transient deformation of cell membranes by EMF indicates a possibility of cellular injury with greater potential damage over longer periods of exposure.[7]

Many studies have focused on the cellular effects of EMF on the brain, likely due to concern of the close proximity of an EMF radiation source to the brain during cell phone use. One study determined that brain tissue will release calcium ions when exposed to weak EMF signals.[8] This calcium release is frequency-specific.[9] The brain's calcium permeability is important because calcium ions help a cell membrane maintain its stability. Insufficient calcium in the cell will weaken the membrane, potentially increasing its permeability.[10] The brain depends on restricted permeability in order to help create a blood-brain barrier, an important defense protecting the brain from pathogens and toxins. Without an intact blood-brain barrier, psychiatric disturbances and neurological diseases such as epilepsy can occur.

Health effects of EMF have been extensively researched throughout the world. Many effects remain controversial. For example, in one study, EMF emitted by a 900-MHz cell phone caused thyroid suppression as documented by abnormal blood tests, including an increased serum thyroid-stimulating hormone (TSH) level, and decreased thyroxine (T4) levels.[11] A different study, performed on rats in Turkey, however, demonstrated that thyroid stimulation by EMF radiation caused a decrease in TSH, T3, and T4 levels.[12]

The EMF radiation emitted by laptops and cell phones has been linked to decreased sperm quality and infertility in men.[13] Placing a cell phone that is turned on and not in airplane mode in a front pocket is not a good idea. A recent scientific paper showed that exposure to 2.45-GHz WiFi for just two hours a day will decrease male fertility.[14] If you are trying to conceive, this is worth knowing.

There have also been many studies that have suggested an association between EMF exposure and cancer.[15,16] As a result of this research, in 2002 and again in 2011, the International Agency for Research on Cancer (IARC), which is a component of the World Health Organization, classified ELF-EMF exposure as possibly carcinogenic to humans (Group 2B).[17]

EMF exposure has been associated with physiological changes of the brain. EMF radiation has been shown to reduce melatonin production by the pineal gland.[18] Studies have shown that the brain "reacts" to RF. Areas of the brain located close to a cell phone's location "light up" on PET scans, indicating that these cells have increased their metabolic rate.[19]

Could EMF exposure be contributing to "brain fog" or some subtle form of dementia or confusion? There is epidemiological evidence that "electropollution" may cause insomnia, daytime tiredness, lack of concentration, memory loss, irritability, and depression.[20,21] Tinnitus (noise or ringing in the ears) has been linked to EMF exposure, but not consistently.[22] The WHO does not recognize a connection between EMF and neurodegenerative diseases, but there are epidemiological studies that suggest EMF may be contributing to the development of neurodegenerative disorders such as ALS, MS, and Parkinson's disease.[23] Scientific experimental studies have not been able to define this relationship.[24]

Many have also questioned whether or not the frequent exposure to this form of radiation, particularly through cell phone use, could cause portions of the brain in closer proximity to the device to have an increased risk of developing cancer. Unfortunately, the literature is contaminated by industry-funded sham research and other badly designed studies overstating or understating the effects of EMF and it is difficult to distill useful information. One study conducted in thirteen countries and organized by the World Health Organization, called the Interphone Study, showed no increase in the incidence of benign brain tumors such as gliomas, acoustic neuromas or meningiomas, or parotid gland (the salivary gland in your cheek) tumors from cell phone use.[25] But in this study, "regular mobile phone users" included all people who used their phone at least once a week for a period of six months. This large range would statistically dilute the data and hide any potential negative effects of the technology. Certainly, those people who use their cell phones or other devices for several hours a day would have a different exposure rate and therefore likely a different risk for developing cancer. High-usage individuals should have been put into a different group than people who use their phone once a week. The diluted study data blurred any potential association between cell phone use and cancer, and concluded that there is no significant increase in cancer incidence in cell phone users. The Interphone Study was partly funded by cell phone companies.

Although the Interphone study did not uncover an overall increase in the development of brain tumors, it did find that benign brain tumors, such as gliomas and meningiomas, were more commonly located on the same side of the head that people held their cell phones against. Other studies have found an increase in the incidence of brain tumors in cell phone users.[26] A more recent study performed by Dr. Lennart Hardell found that tumor growth occurred many years after exposure, a delay called the latency period. The average latency period in his study was nine years. But the most significant increase in tumors developed after a latency period of more than fifteen years.[27]

In children, the effects of EMF radiation are particularly worrisome. Pooled data analyzed from many independent studies performed in several different countries documented a twofold increase in leukemia risk in children with the highest exposure to ELF-EMF.[28] There is a good reason why the European Assembly passed Resolution 1815, which restricts the use of WiFi in schools and restricts the use of mobile phones by children. The question is: Why don't we have similar restrictions here in the US? Our governmental agencies, including the National Institutes of Health (NIH), the Federal Communications Commission (FCC), and the Centers for Disease Control and Prevention (CDC), assert there is no conclusive link between cell phone use and any adverse health problems, but these agencies do agree that more research is needed.

"EMF toxicity" is not a concept that many scientists are willing to acknowledge. Regardless, there are groups of people who have come to the conclusion that their poor health is the direct result of electropollution and that the only "cure" for them has been to remove all sources of EMF radiation from their environment. In extreme cases, people have needed to move to remote locations where there are no EMF frequencies being generated or received. Although only a very small subset of people appears to have a severe "allergy" to EMF radiation, it has been suggested that all people are affected in some way or another by EMF, even though most people don't ascribe their symptoms to electropollution. Most physicians are only trained to explore anatomical or biochemical abnormalities that could explain a patient's symptoms. Vertigo and tinnitus are common symptoms for people who suffer from electropollution, but most patients and physicians are not ready to explore their link to EMF. Instead, patients undergo expensive diagnostic imaging studies and lab testing to uncover potential structural abnormalities causing these ethereal symptoms. But knowing that the brain is a conductor of electrochemical impulses, is it a stretch to consider that environmental EMF currents could have an effect on the nervous system?

The symptoms attributed to electrosensitivity are numerous and controversial, ranging from headaches and tinnitus to asthma attacks, muscular weakness, and acne. Physicians may label a patient with these types of symptoms as a hypochondriac if all of the testing results are normal. Even though most people have no clinical symptoms related to EMF, the cellular effects are most likely the same for everyone. Some people, however, are more sensitive to this form of energy than others. Regardless of whether or not one can sense EMF, it has been suggested that frequent exposure to it causes the body to age faster than its genetic programming. Whether this is a result of decreased melatonin production or direct damage to the cell membranes or DNA is uncertain.

Detecting EMF

So what does one do with this information? First, it is necessary to identify the sources of electropollution within and around your home. Although EMF cannot be discerned with the ears or other senses, there are detectors that will find sources of EMF and quantify its intensity. An EMF detector is not a major purchase. A high-frequency detector is the most versatile meter for EMF assessment in the home and will cost around $300. With the EMF detector in hand, walk around your home, aiming the detector toward the walls, ceiling, and floor. The detector will click and produce noises along with a numerical display corresponding to the strength of the EMF signal.

The more common sources of EMF radiation found in and around the typical American home are listed in Table 10.

Table 10. EMF sources in the typical home

Cordless phone	Computer games
Neighbor's house	Cell phone
Tablet computers	Nearby cell phone tower
Microwave oven	Baby monitors
WiFi router	Smart meters
Car key fob	Wireless security systems

When moving through your home with a detector, pick a distance from which you want to monitor the strength of emissions from each EMF source. In our home, we chose a distance of six feet and made a chart listing the readings obtained from each source. This gave us a sense of how strong each emission is. Keep in mind that your exposure to the radiation from each source will vary depending on your location and distance from the device. For example, your cordless phone may be located only two or three feet from your head while you sleep at night if it sits on a nightstand next to the bed. Similarly, if you are in the kitchen and your portable phone is on the counter next to you, it may be less than four feet from you as you stand making dinner or washing dishes. The intensity of EMF, similar to all other forms of radiation, follows an inverse square law, meaning that the intensity of the radiation will be proportional to the square of the distance you are from the source. So, if you double your distance from the source of emission, say, by moving from six feet to twelve feet, the exposure at twelve feet will be one-quarter what it was at six feet. In addition to jotting down the maximum intensity of each source at a specified distance, note whether the radiation is a continuous or intermittent source of EMF. After this process, it is time to think about remediation.

Remediation

Depending on the sources and the intensity of EMF in the home, remediation may be simple or complex. All forms of radiation dissipate over distance, so the greater the distance between you and each source of radiation, the better for your health. In addition to increasing distance from each radiation source, the creation of energy-reflecting or absorption barriers between the home occupants and each

EMF source is another way to limit exposure. This technique, referred to as shielding, can be achieved by applying specific types of paint, fabric, screening material, etc. Shielding material provides a highly conductive path for the EMF to travel along, limiting its dispersion. There are many different types of shielding fabrics available, and they can be used to form curtains, canopies for the bed, clothing, bedding, wall coverings, etc.

Another suggested method for reducing the effects of EMF on the body is grounding oneself to the earth. This process, called earthing, has been shown to equalize electrical potentials between the body and the earth, effectively canceling, reducing, or pushing away electric fields. It has been suggested that the absence of grounding may be one of the contributing factors to developing symptoms of electropollution. The easiest way to ground oneself is to walk barefoot or in leather-soled shoes. Earthing mats are said to provide grounding when they are plugged into the grounding outlets of electrical sockets. Unfortunately, most electrical outlets contain a "dirty electricity" that can flow back through the wire and affect the body. So, unless there is a filter to clean the electricity emanating from the outlet, many don't recommend this method of grounding.

Common EMF emitters

WiFi router

If an EMF detector is directed toward a wireless router, it will sound like a jackhammer twenty-four hours a day. A WiFi router should be placed as far away from living spaces as possible. A bedroom is not an appropriate place for a router, where it could be detrimental to one's health, for the person trying to relax and sleep in the room will be constantly bombarded with EMF. It would be prudent to move the router to the basement or another room far away from where you sleep. If the router cannot be moved far enough away to significantly reduce the EMF exposure in living spaces, turn it off when it is not in use. In addition, placing the router on an electric timer that will automatically turn it off at night and back on in the morning can work well.

Cordless phones

Cordless phones are convenient, but they can emit a large amount of EMF. The systems that produce the most EMF are those with multiple remote handsets. The base station emits an EMF beacon signal a hundred times per second to maintain contact with the remote handsets. If you must have a cordless phone, choose one that doesn't constantly radiate EMF, such as the ECO-DECT II. Better yet, remove the cordless phones and, in their place, position a few corded landline telephones. They typically cost under ten dollars apiece and do not emit any EMF.

Cell phones

All cell phones emit EMF when they are sending and receiving data. Smart phones emit EMF not only when you talk or text, but also when you receive pushed notifications, messages, and emails. If a cell phone is idle and not in use, it will most likely emit a strong, periodic ping.

Try to keep your smart phone as far away from your body while it is turned on, even when it isn't in use. Carry the phone in a jacket pocket, carrying bag, or knapsack. If a smart phone is turned off or placed in airplane mode, it should not emit any EMF radiation.

When making a voice call, one should not press a cell phone up against the ear. Cell phone instructions specify to maintain a distance between the phone and skin surface while the phone is in use. The iPhone 4 booklet specifies a distance of 5/8", which is probably still too close. Medical imaging studies have circulated around the Internet showing localized heating of the brain from cell phone EMF, which can occur after only a few minutes of cell phone use. This heating effect is even more significant in children, probably due to their thinner skulls. Try to limit your child's cell phone use and delay it as long as possible. Instruct your children to never put the phone in their pockets or to hold the phone up to their heads.

Bluetooth wireless devices reportedly deliver around a hundred times less EMF than a typical mobile phone, which sounds significant. But consider that even 1/100th the EMF radiation of a cell phone is still higher than what is considered acceptable for a background level of EMF. Both Bluetooth devices and earbuds placed in the ear provide a short, direct passageway for the EMF to travel through the ear and into the brain, and through the internal auditory canal where the auditory and vestibular cranial nerves are located. These nerves are more commonly associated with the benign tumors known as schwannoma and acoustic neuroma.

When using a cell phone for a voice call, use the speaker function or use a "blue tube" device to give you more privacy. The blue tube is a safer device than Bluetooth. In this apparatus, the wiring ends approximately a foot from the earbud, and a hollow, flexible tube transmits the sound from the wire up into the ear. EMF radiation does not get transmitted into the ear. Blue tubes can also come with EMF shields. Device shields are becoming popular for use with cell phones as well as with other wireless devices.

Tablets, iPods, etc.

Although they are called "laptops," these devices should not put on a lap unless there is a protective shield beneath the unit to block EMF emissions. Pregnant women should be especially careful not to place a tablet, laptop, or iPod on their stomachs with WiFi turned on, as this will subject the unborn child to strong EMF fields. Neuronal migration in the developing brain relies on subtle electromagnetic currents in the fetus, which could potentially be distorted by the exogenous EMF emitted by a wireless device. There are dozens of magnetic shields available for use with wireless devices. Do a little investigation and see which one will work best for you.

Microwave ovens

I never really cared for the uneven heating so common with microwave ovens, and after evaluating the oven for EMF emission, we removed the unit from the house. If you prefer to cook meals with a microwave, test the oven when it is operating and see if there is any EMF leakage. If there is, see how far the radiation travels. In our home, the EMF emitted by the microwave oven radiated through the wall and all the way across the adjacent living room. If your oven leaks EMF, there are a few options. If you replace the unit, check the new unit with the EMF detector to make sure the new one doesn't leak. Alternatively, you can leave the area of radiation exposure while the unit is operating. The most preferable option, in my opinion, is to select a different method for heating your food and water.

Computer games

Wii consoles, Sony PlayStations, and other game consoles emit significantly less EMF than those devices that utilize WiFi. Regardless, when finished with these games, it is easy to unplug the console. Try to avoid playing these games before bedtime, as EMF emissions from devices can affect melatonin production, as with other WiFi-enabled devices.

Baby monitors

It's been a long time since we've had a baby in the house, but I do remember those nights as a nervous father, wondering if the baby was doing all right while we were lying in the bedroom next door, in the darkness. Baby monitors allow a parent to hear every breath, gurgle, and cry that the baby may utter when the parent or guardian is in another room. But baby monitors produce a constant emission of EMF radiation. Check the emission strength with an EMF detector and see if you can place the monitor at a distance close enough that you can hear the baby, but far enough away that the baby is not receiving a high dose of EMF radiation. If this is not possible because the EMF pulse is too strong, or because the room is too small, try partially wrapping the monitor in magnetic shielding foil, or making an EMF blockade with shielding material or foil. Sound will travel around the shielding material, but EMF will be blocked.

Electric blankets

Electric blankets emit EMF. As electricity travels through the wiring in the blanket, heat and an electromagnetic field are generated. As there is no barrier between your skin and either the electrical field or the magnetic field, much has been written about whether or not this is a safe source of heat. Early research suggested that exposure to high levels of EMF, such as from an electric blanket, slightly increased the risk of miscarriage[29,30] and so the recommendation was that pregnant women should not use electric blankets during the first or third trimesters of pregnancy. Many subsequent studies, though, have shown there to be no increased risk of miscarriage from electric blankets.[31]

Although research shows that EMF fields may not be severe enough to cause miscarriages, it seems possible that non-fatal, damaging effects might occur to the developing fetal brain, which undergoes a process called neural migration during pregnancy. Until further research is conducted and our knowledge of this sensitive time is more complete, I would recommend not using an electric blanket at all during pregnancy.

Dirty electricity

Dirty electricity is a term given to high-frequency noise over 1 kHz that mixes in with your home's electrical current. Dirty electricity is mostly created by devices within your home, but it can also travel into your home from your electricity supplier. Dirty electricity is a relatively small source of EMF as compared to other sources, but for one who is EMF sensitive, the use of a dirty electricity filter may help reduce the quantity of emissions and may abate symptoms of EMF toxicity. One brand, Greenware, makes filters that plug into existing outlets and help filter out electrical noise before it has a chance to radiate into the room. One to 3 filter plugs are needed per room, depending on the amount of electronics within that room.

Exterior sources of EMF

Given the technological advances of wireless communication, it is no surprise that the industry has developed meters that are able to tell your utility company how much usage you have registered without the need for an employee to come to your home to look at the utility meter. These "smart meters" report back to the company, divulging information about your energy usage throughout the day, every day. When you check your walls, make sure to aim the EMF detector at the interior wall space behind the smart meter's location on your home exterior.

EMF radiation originating from outside your home may also come from your neighbor's home, a local cell phone tower, or a nearby power line. Your ability to decrease your family's exposure to exogenous EMF radiation is dependent on how well you shield your home from radiation sources.

If EMF is coming through a wall, a specialized paint designed to reflect EMF can be applied to the interior wall. In addition to paints, fabrics and plates can be applied. These reflective materials need to be grounded by a professional electrician. If the EMF is coming through a window, treat the window's interior with clear reflective window coatings, which will effectively shield the RF pulse. If none of these alternatives are feasible, a specialized shielding canopy can be suspended from the ceiling and spread out to surround a bed. These canopies will protect one from EMF while sleeping. During the daytime, if one is exposed to a significant amount of unavoidable EMF, clothing specially designed to reflect EMF radiation may be helpful.

In conclusion

Numerous sources of EMF are found in the typical home. Reducing strong EMF emissions from WiFi, portable phones, microwave ovens, etc. will help to create a more relaxed atmosphere and may improve the overall health of all living in the home.

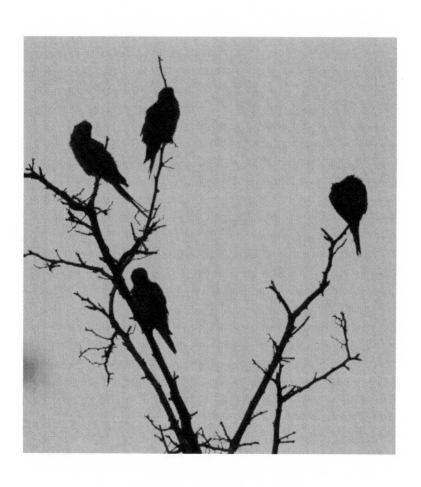

Chapter 10
LIGHT

Imagine living in a world without artificial sources of light. As the sun rises, you become filled with energy. You spend the day aware and alert. As the sun begins to set, you settle down to end the day, perhaps becoming contemplative. As the skies darken, you prepare for slumber. As darkness covers the sky, the body is ready to sleep and your mind shifts into a sleep mode. The body repairs itself while the mind reorganizes and attempts to solve problems encountered during the day through dreams.

To get a sense of life without artificial light, go camping. Sleep in a tent for a few nights, away from all sources of artificial light, except for maybe a flashlight. People who camp and rise with the sun often go to sleep not long after the sun sets. People with sleep disturbances will commonly have their sleep patterns stabilize if taken on camping trips.

Even though we live in a world filled with artificial light, hormonal effects, mood effects, and sleep disturbances seem to be associated with the phases of the moon.[1] I have spoken with several physicians and nurses who acknowledge that their emergency rooms are busier and people more agitated, nervous, and sicker during full moons. Teachers and educators have commented to me that their students are more out of control during the full moon. Throughout my years of work, I have noticed that diseases such as congestive failure seem to be exacerbated during full moons. This observation was first described by Hippocrates, and continues to be an unexplained curiosity even today. However, many research studies have not been able to confirm this phenomenon. If these effects are related to the moon's phases and luminosity, could it be that the effects are obscured in cities and larger towns with increased light pollution?

Sight is possible because our eyes are able to extract information from a thin band of electromagnetic energy called the visible light spectrum. Light enters the eye through the cornea, a clear protective covering that prevents the passage of air and debris into the eye. Light then passes through the lens, where it is focused and directed through a hole in the iris called the pupil. The iris is a dynamic structure that will open and close depending on light intensity. In bright light, the iris constricts, diminishing the size of the pupil. In darkness, the iris relaxes and dilates, allowing more light to come in. Once light passes through the pupil, it travels through a thick, gelatinous, clear material called vitreous fluid which fills the majority of the globe and gives it a round shape. Finally, focused light hits the back wall of the eye, known as the retina, which is composed of specialty cells that are able to convert light into electrical impulses. This signal is transmitted through the optic nerve to the brain where it is decoded in the visual cortex. Neural pathways in the brain connect the visual cortex to other areas of the brain and allow cognition and associative memory to identify and understand what we see.

Visible light consists of a thin band of wavelengths between 400 and 780 nm, situated between infrared (IR) and ultraviolet (UV) wavelengths in the electromagnetic spectrum (Figure 1). IR wavelengths are between 780 nm and 1 mm and are further sub-classified into IRA, IRB, and IRC. IRA is the frequency nearest to visible light. UV wavelengths are shorter, between 100 and 400 nm. UV radiation is sub-classified into UVA, UVB, and UVC wavelengths, with UVA being closest to visible light.

Figure 4. The electromagnetic spectrum

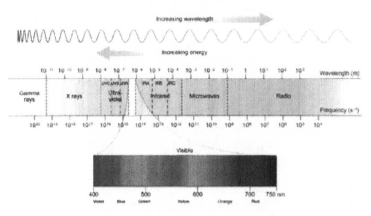

Why is this relevant? It is important to understand that when we are placed into light, we are exposed to a broader range of wavelengths than what we can see with our eyes. Light sources produce bands of wavelength that far exceed the visible light spectrum. Humans can detect IR wavelengths by feeling the heat they generate. UV wavelengths do not produce heat and cannot be "sensed" by the body, but they can damage skin.

The sun produces frequencies throughout the electromagnetic spectrum. By the time the sun's energy reaches the Earth's atmosphere, however, the remaining wavelengths are in the range from IR to UV. The atmosphere effectively blocks most of the UV and IR radiation from reaching the earth's surface, protecting us from most of the sun's harmful rays. The sunlight that reaches us is a white light, composed of an equal distribution of wavelengths across the visible light spectrum. It is a full-spectrum light, meaning it has a broad, flat, spectral power distribution (SPD).

Light physiology

Aside from providing us with an ability to see, the retina contains receptors that respond to light, independent of the visual system's rods and cones. These receptors send information about the presence or absence of light directly to a different section of the brain called the suprachiasmatic nucleus (SCN), located within the hypothalamus. By sensing light and dark, our bodies can become synchronized to the movement of the Earth's rotation and its orbit around the sun. Although the SCN receives input from other stimuli, the most potent stimulus for our synchronization to the twenty-four-hour day/night cycle is through the temporal exposure to light. Wavelengths between 460 and 484 nm (blue light) have been shown to be the most effective at stimulating these retinal cells.[2] Light therefore enables us to see and also provides us with a mechanism with which we can generate a biological clock, known as a circadian rhythm, which syncs our bodies to the Earth's rotation and orbit.

By closing our eyes, it is possible to "turn off" one's visual system. However, dropping the eyelids is not an effective way to stop light from entering the eye. Eyelids are merely a protective mechanism that keep our eyes moist, help wipe away debris, and allow us a way to turn off visual sensory input. However, depending on the intensity of ambient light, closing one's eyes may be akin to putting non-blackout curtains on an outdoor window during a sunny day. Napping in a room with ambient light will more than likely stimulate the SCN, telling the body that it is daytime.

Melatonin

Why does this matter? A small gland in the brain, called the pineal gland, is also connected to the SCN. If the pineal gland receives information through the SCN pathway that indicates it is nighttime, it will produce and release the hormone N-acetyl-5-methoxytryptamine, also called melatonin, into the bloodstream. Interestingly, the pineal gland has been referred to as the third eye in many cultures for thousands of years. By responding to light via the SCN pathway, it does, in a sense, act like an eye, although it sends the brain no spatial information and can't stimulate any associative memories.

The pineal gland commonly becomes partially calcified as we age, as often seen on CT exams. Although many think this calcification does not appear to have any effect on the pineal gland's function, one study found an association between pineal calcification and a loss of directional sense.[3] The pineal gland's release of melatonin has significant effects on the brain and on maintaining the body's overall health. Melatonin is synthesized during sleep in the darkness of night, with peak production usually around 2 am, both during the summer and winter.[4] Circadian rhythm is therefore timed to a cyclical production of melatonin during darkness and non-production during periods of light. Melatonin provides the cells in our body with a chemical biological clock that indicates to the body's systems the length of the night and signals the brain as to when it is dusk and dawn. Longer nights during winter result in greater melatonin secretion, and shorter nights during summer result in less melatonin production.[5] In this way, our bodies can differentiate between the seasons.

Melatonin has important physiological effects. Higher levels (longer nights, deeper sleep) strengthen the immune system, while lower levels (shorter nights and/or interrupted sleep) suppress a number of immune system actions.[6] Melatonin is a powerful antioxidant and functions as an anti-cancer agent by interacting directly with cancer cells.[7] Melatonin also affects the production and release of proteins such as reproductive hormones,[8] which may directly or indirectly affect cancer growth. Melatonin has also been shown to be an epigenetic regulator, meaning that the presence or absence of melatonin in a cell can determine which genes in the DNA are switched on and off.[9] Abnormal melatonin levels are commonly encountered in a number of psychiatric and neurological disorders, including depression.[10]

Melatonin is an important hormone that ties us to our environment, strengthens our immune systems, and even affects our genetic expression. So, what happens when melatonin production goes haywire? First, consider why melatonin production might be insufficient. As mentioned earlier, melatonin production ceases when the pineal gland senses light. Exposure to a room light in the evening, before bedtime, has also been shown to have a profound suppressing effect on melatonin production.[11] Even viewing a lit LED screen before going to sleep has been shown to significantly lower melatonin levels and suppress sleep.[12] The effect is more profound in children and teenagers than in adults. In fact, the degree of melatonin suppression caused by nighttime light exposure in children is almost twice that for adults.[13] Blue light suppresses melatonin to a greater extent than longer wavelengths (redder colors).[2] Insomnia can be attributed in some cases to decreased melatonin production, particularly in the elderly.[14] Perhaps this may sometimes be related to elderly people falling asleep with the television on, or perhaps not being able to fully close their eyes while they are sleeping.

Studies have indicated that exposure to low levels of artificial light in the home or office during the day and/or increased light at night may disturb melatonin production and therefore disrupt circadian rhythms.[15] We are designed to be exposed to sunlight during the day and darkness at night— otherwise, we can become out of sync and lose our circadian rhythms.

Disrupted circadian rhythms caused by light exposure at night have been associated with sleep, gastrointestinal, mood, and cardiovascular disorders, possibly through diminished melatonin production.[16] There is epidemiological evidence that disrupted circadian rhythms and insufficient melatonin production have caused an increased incidence of breast cancer in:

> Night shift workers. Women who do long term shift work have a 40% increased risk of developing breast cancer![17]
> Flight attendants potentially suffering from jet lag and night shift work.[18]
> Increased ambient light at night in the bedroom.[19]
> Increased light in the community at night (light pollution).[20]

Additional studies show that cancer risk in general increases with deficient melatonin, meaning that if one's circadian rhythms are disrupted, one is at risk for developing many other different types of cancer.[21]

So what should you do if you are stuck with a job where you are required to do overnight work? Quit? Limiting the number of people required to work graveyard shifts throughout the workforce would indeed lead to benefits in society's overall health.

For those who are not required to work graveyard shifts, there are several lifestyle changes that can help maintain normal melatonin production and balanced circadian rhythms.

First of all, pick a bedtime, ideally before 1 am, and try to stick with it. When your body senses it is time to go to sleep, it will naturally produce hormones that prepare your body for sleep. If you fight this urge, you may find that your sleepiness will dissipate and you will then have a hard time falling asleep later.

If you like to read before bed, choose your reading light carefully. Consider using a small spot-type LED light that will illuminate your book pages, but not the room. Tablets and computers should not be viewed in bed prior to sleeping, especially by teenagers. The TV should be turned off when you go to sleep. If needed, put a timer on the TV to have it automatically shut off at a specified time, soon after you anticipate falling asleep.

Make sure your bedroom is dark. Many electronic gadgets are equipped with LED indicator lights that faintly glow in the darkness of the bedroom. Put black tape over them or place an object in front of each indicator light so you can't see them with your eyes open. Studies have shown that even periodic, faint flashes of light in an otherwise dark bedroom can delay and diminish melatonin secretion,[22] even if the sleeper does not awaken. If you have an alarm clock with a lighted display, dim the display or turn it off. If you live in an area with light pollution, purchase blackout blinds or curtains. When the window treatment is closed, no exterior light should enter the room.

If these suggestions are not possible, an eye mask can help. These products typically consist of a soft fabric overlying a sponge-like insert with elastic straps. Some masks are filled with lavender or other herbs. It may initially be difficult sleeping with a mask on, but after a few nights, you will more than likely find it easier to fall asleep with them on and your nights will be more restful.

In most cases, modifications to one's lifestyle should restore normal melatonin levels. If not, though, a melatonin supplement can be used. Melatonin supplements are produced and marketed as sleep enhancers and treatments for depression and jet lag. Many additional applications for melatonin supplementation exist. Even people taking statins have been shown to benefit from melatonin supplementation as melatonin has a protective effect on the liver.[23] No significant side effects are associated with the use of melatonin.[24]

Excessive melatonin production can occur in people who do not get enough light exposure, as can happen during winter months in the northern latitudes.[25] Too much darkness or insufficient daylight exposure can cause seasonal affective disorder (SAD),[26] a condition resulting from the overproduction of melatonin. Many of us who go to work before the sun rises, stay indoors all day, and then leave work as the sun sets are well aware of how the winter months slowly drag by as we get more and more glum. Regardless of one's job, it is important to take time every day to bathe in outdoor light. Even on cloudy days, going outside into daylight, even if it is just for ten minutes, will improve your mood and well-being. SAD can be successfully treated without medication by administering daily light "therapy."[27]

Interior lighting

Because we have created opaque housing to live in and lifestyles that carry us into the night, we have a need for interior lighting. The most common method for providing light to an interior space is to create a window that allows the sun's light to enter, known as daylighting. During periods of insufficient daylight, the need for indoor light production is apparent. In many parts of the world today, people rely on fire for indoor light. In other parts of the world where electricity is readily accessible, indoor lighting is achieved through light bulbs, referred to in the industry as lamps.

Lamps are evaluated for their SPD, the assessment of emission at each wavelength in the visible light spectrum. This analysis is used to determine three unique qualities for each lamp, including color temperature, color rendering index, and light intensity. These qualities determine the overall color appearance of the light. Natural daylight has a broad, flat SPD and is thought by many to be best for health and well-being.

A light's brightness or intensity is measured in lumens. A lumen is a standard unit corresponding to the amount of light generated by one candle flame. For comparison, daylight intensity is on the order of 50,000-100,000 lumens. Lamps with higher wattage provide brighter, more intense light.

Light's color temperature is measured in the Kelvin (K) scale. Noon daylight is a white light with a corresponding temperature of approximately 5500K. Light bulbs that appear more reddish have a lower temperature than bulbs that are bluer in color. A typical warm (reddish) white fluorescent lamp may have a color temperature of 3000K while a cool white fluorescent bulb (more bluish) may have a temperature of 4100K. This is the opposite of what one might expect—the warmly-colored, reddish bulb is cooler in temperature than the cool-colored blue bulb.

The color rendering index (CRI) is an assessment of how close in color objects appear within an artificial light source as compared to their appearance in natural daylight. Outdoor light has a perfect CRI of 100 by definition. A lamp with a CRI of 80 will show colors more naturally than a lamp with a CRI of 60. The CRI for most fluorescent bulbs ranges between 60 and 75. This light characteristic is important because not only do objects such as food and skin look more normal in a room illuminated with a high CRI lamp, this quality light allows us to see detail more clearly, with less eye fatigue and strain than do lower CRI bulbs.[28]

When choosing how to provide light to the interior of your home, start by daylighting as much as possible through the installation of windows and sky lights. During the night hours and in rooms with limited natural light, lamps are needed.

The categories of electrically produced artificial light include incandescent lamps, halogen lamps, electrical discharge lamps, LEDs, and other forms of solid-state lighting. Each product uses a different technology to produce the light. There are pros and cons to each type of lamp, and some are potentially more toxic than others.

Incandescent lamps are those lights bulbs that illuminate by passing electricity through a metal filament until the filament glows. As the temperature rises, so does the wavelength of the light, thereby changing the color temperature of the light. Incandescent bulbs produce IR radiation, emitting heat as well as light. Higher-frequency bulbs produce a blue light and some UV radiation, but the levels of UV radiation are not thought to be significant.[29]

Halogen bulbs are similar to incandescent lamps in that the electrical current travels through a filament, but the filament is located in a chamber filled with a halogen gas so it can get very hot without melting. These bulbs are more efficient than incandescent bulbs and they produce a brighter light, closer to natural daylight. Because of the intense heat these bulbs produce, they need to be placed in special fixtures. Because bare halogen bulbs emit a significant amount of UVA, UVB, and UVC radiation, these bulbs are usually placed within a coated envelope to increase their safety. The coating, applied to the glass interior, filters out UV radiation. Sometimes these bulbs are placed within a second glass envelope, further reducing radiation. Treated bulbs do still emit low levels of UVA, UVB, and UVC radiation.[30]

Electrical discharge lamps do not have a filament and instead produce light by sending an electrical current through a gas. This category of lighting includes fluorescent bulbs. The color and intensity of the light produced depends on the pressure and the type of gas within the bulb. There are many variations in this type of lamp, with only a few types suitable for indoor home use. Fluorescent lights are composed of a glass tube, the inside of which is coated with phosphor, and filled with low- pressure mercury vapor. As current passes through the vapor, it creates UV radiation, causing the phosphor layer to glow and create visible white light. Compact fluorescent lamps fall into this category and have largely replaced incandescent bulbs, as they are much more efficient.

Compact fluorescent lamp bulbs

Compact fluorescent lamp bulbs (CFLs) became the main light source for people living in the US after incandescent bulbs were phased out at the beginning of 2014. CFLs were first introduced in the 1970s and went through many variations. These bulbs need time to warm up to reach full brightness. They are filled with various gases, including argon, mercury vapor, tungsten, barium, strontium, and calcium oxides. It is the mercury vapor that has many people alarmed about their safety. A CFL typically contains 5 mg of mercury, which is 1/100th of the amount of mercury that used to be inside the old-style thermometer.[31] In the event of bulb breakage, only a small fraction of that mercury is released into the air. A 2011 study showed that a broken bulb released less than 4% of the mercury contained within it into the air. However, the bulbs continue to emit mercury vapor into the air for up to ten weeks after breaking.[32] After a few days, the amount of mercury gas emitted from a broken bulb can exceed 1 milligram, exceeding what the EPA considers safe for children.[33] A safe cleanup is recommended in order to minimize exposure. According to the EPA, the following steps, listed on their website, are required to safely clean up a broken CFL bulb (Figure 5).

Figure 5. Broken CFL bulb clean-up

1. Have people and pets leave the room.
2. Air out the room for 5-10 minutes by opening up a window or door to the outside.
3. Shut off central forced air heat or air conditioning.
4. Collect materials for cleanup:
    Stiff piece of paper or cardboard Sticky tape
    Damp paper towel or disposable wipes
    A glass jar with a metal lid or a sealable plastic bag
5. Do not vacuum!
6. Use paper or cardboard to scoop up glass fragments and any visible powder
7. Use sticky tape to pick up any residual powder.
8. Place the cardboard, paper and any used tape in the glass jar or plastic bag and seal.
9. Bring all clean up materials outdoors to a trash can/bin. Don't leave any used cleaning materials inside.
10. Check with local municipality/government about disposal requirements.
11. Leave heating/air conditioning off for several hours.

If you print out this list and keep it along with some tape, paper towels, a sealable plastic bag, and a piece of cardboard in the cabinet where you keep extra light bulbs, you will be ready for clean-up in the event you have a broken bulb. As mentioned in #9, don't leave any clean-up materials indoors. Mercury vapors can penetrate through plastic bags.[33]

Most CFL bulbs have defects that allow UV radiation to leak from them at levels potentially damaging to skin.[34] Many CFL bulbs emit UVB radiation that is above the occupational exposure limit at 25 cm, set by the American conference of Governmental Industrial Hygienists. Although UVC is also emitted by some bulbs, this wavelength of UV radiation does not extend more than 10 cm beyond the bulb.[35]

CFL bulbs may be a single envelope, with an exposed spiral loop, or a double envelope, with a second layer of protective glass placed around the spiral gas-filled loop. People with skin diseases who are sensitive to UVA may react to bulbs with a second glass envelope, as these bulbs do sometimes emit UVA at levels that can exacerbate symptoms.[36] Some medications and personal care products, such as tetracycline, antidepressants, diuretics, antipsychotics, and certain cosmetics, can make people hypersensitive to UV light. In order to protect yourself from the potential toxicity associated with CFL bulbs, place bulbs inside a fixture, use them in a well-ventilated room, and keep them at least twenty inches away from the room occupant while it is turned on. These are not appropriate bulbs to use as night lights or for close-up detail or desk work.

Full-spectrum fluorescent lights (FSFLs) produce the full spectral power distribution range (both visible and UV) of natural outdoor light. FSFLs have been credited by some to cause dramatic beneficial health effects, including improved cognition and perception. However, no reproducible association between FSFLs and human wellness has been effectively documented.

Light-emitting diodes (LEDs) produce light through electroluminescence. These lights have become very popular because they are safer and more efficient than CFLs. These lights are typically colored, but full-spectrum LED lights contain multiple colors that produce white light when combined. LED lights are, in general, a safe and efficient light source, but they do contain arsenic, copper, nickel, and lead. The amount of each depends on the color and brand of the bulb.

Which bulbs and where?

With so many lamp types and wattages to choose from, it is important to consider the light intensity and color spectrum optimal for each room. Insufficient light and over-illumination can both be undesirable. Examine each room in the home and decide which type of lighting is desired in each space. Choose between three basic categories: ambient lighting, accent lighting, and task lighting.

The most common type of room lighting, ambient lighting, includes those lighting fixtures that illuminate a whole room, such as overhead lights, floor lamps, and table lamps. For this purpose, CFLs and LEDs are both suitable and efficient options. The fixtures will be far enough from people in the room that CFLs should not cause any hazardous effects with the small amount of UV radiation or gas they emit.

Accent lighting is intended to be more decorative and can be used to highlight pictures, plants, or other elements of interior design. When aiming a light source at a piece of artwork, it is very important to consider the frailty of the media. Certainly, watercolors, gouaches, and other media that can fade need to be kept out of direct sunlight and also away from full-spectrum lights and CFLs. LED bulbs are most suitable for displaying artwork. Oil paintings are inherently more stable than watercolors and can be exposed to direct sunlight and all types of light bulbs. Plants thrive under full-spectrum fluorescent and LED lights. Blue light is optimal for plant growth and when combined with red light, flowering and fruiting are promoted.[37] CFLs and LEDs run cool in temperature, provide a broad-spectrum light, and can function as grow lights. Halogen and incandescent bulbs usually run too hot to be safe for plants. Other forms of accent lighting can include downlighting, uplighting, backlighting, etc. Depending on the esthetic affects you want to achieve in your room, the source and direction of light can be used to create different moods and atmospheres. LED lights have become the popular choice for this effect.

Task lighting should aid one in reading and inspecting close-up details. CFLs are not recommended for these tasks. Halogen bulbs produce bright white light and make a more suitable light for close-up detail work. If you are light sensitive, however, LED lighting would be an even better choice for task lighting. Home office lighting should be bright and have increased blue frequency. Blue lights and white light artificially enriched with blue frequency "cool lights" have an enhancing effect on cognition, memory, and mood that is stronger than for warm, reddish lights.[38]

Bedroom lighting choices are especially important. In addition to being a place for sleep, an adult's bedroom is typically a refuge from the daily chaos in a home, and a private location to discuss and evaluate important decisions. An assortment of lighting options in the bedroom is desirable. Both positive and negative human emotions are felt more intensely in bright light,[39] so it is helpful to have ambient lights on a dimmer and to dim the lights when conducting negotiations and making rational decisions. For reading lights, neither bright lights nor CFL bulbs are a good choice as they can affect melatonin production. A focused LED light that will illuminate pages in the book while leaving the rest of the room dark would be ideal for this task.

In summary

Honor the sun when it is in the sky by letting it provide you with as much light as possible during the day and when indoors, choose your light sources carefully. During nighttime, try to limit exposure to full spectrum lights, particularly before bedtime, to ensure you get a good night's rest. In this way, your body will produce adequate melatonin, which will keep your immune system and body in a healthier state.

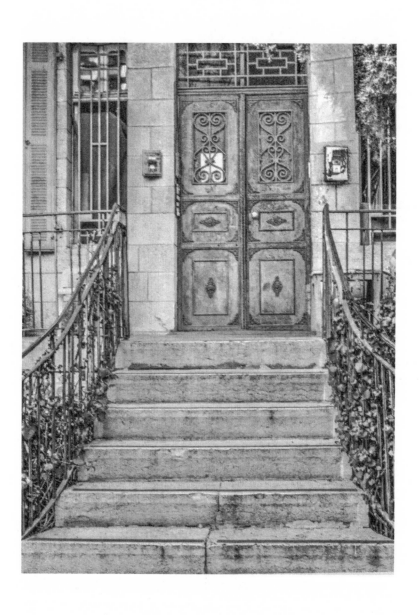

Chapter 11
FENG SHUI

Putting together a living space, arranging furniture, choosing colors for the walls and other decor can provide one with a sense of satisfaction. When people enter your home and say, "Wow, this place feels so comfortable!" it creates a sense of pride in the homeowner. Not every idea works, though, and sometimes one may sense there's something not quite right about the environment. The reason may be obvious, like clutter. At other times, the source may be more subtle and obscure. A room's design can make one feel relaxed or ill at ease, even stressed out. *Feng shui* is the study of energy flow within the home and understanding a bit about this topic will help you create a harmonious home environment.

Feng shui is more abstract than the other types of toxicity this book has been concerned with thus far. It is an ancient discipline, dating back thousands of years, that teaches the practitioner to manipulate the movement of energy. Areas in the home can have flowing energy and areas of stagnation, which, according to Chinese tradition, can be healthy or toxic. To some, this study may seem like superstition or even carry religious connotations because the study of *feng shui* is a natural extension of the *I Ching*, the Chinese book of ancient wisdom and spirituality.

There are many different conceptual schools of practice that fall under the umbrella label "*feng shui*." Regardless of which school is studied, the tools of *feng shui* can be applied to all aspects of one's life. This chapter will introduce basic concepts to help the reader create a positive energy flow into and throughout their home. According to practitioners, belief in the system is not needed for it to work.

Proper energy flow in the home will transfer through to the rest of one's life. If your home is configured properly, you will more likely live a healthy and prosperous life. If it isn't, you may suffer from health, financial, relationship, and/or career misfortune. From my own personal experiences, I do believe that poor energy flow can be toxic to one's well-being.

I have come to understand *feng shui* as an endless search for the achievement of balance. The discipline can be applied to your property and surrounding landscape, in addition to smaller domains, such as the home, rooms in the home, and even the placement of objects within each room. In *feng shui*, one can create a positive energy flow into the home from your property and beyond.

Feng shui translates to "wind and water," two sources of inanimate movement in the natural world. This study involves the methodical capturing of this energy and graciously moving it throughout the home, property, and life. The underlying premise is that everything in the world, and in fact, the universe, is composed of energy, referred to as *chi*. Differing arrangements of the basic elements air, fire, water, wood, and metal can either generate energy, facilitate the movement and flow of energy, or cause energy stagnation and loss. The steering of good energy into the home and the controlled movement of energy throughout one's home is most desirable.

In this system, your home is considered to be a representation and manifestation of your life, and its rooms are therefore symbolic of you and your family. The front door of your home is analogous to the mouth and the windows are symbolic of the eyes. The back of the home is like the back of your home's head and needs to be protected, ideally by a hill or by tall trees. Water and wind that move toward your front door bring you and your home energy, whereas water and wind that move away from your home deplete energy. Bedrooms should be calm, whereas other parts of the home, such as the living room and family room, should be lively. Collecting and manipulating the flow of energy can create a greater state of peace and relaxation in the parts of the home where you need rest, and vitality in parts of the home where activity is needed.

Yin and *yang*

Before learning how to apply *feng shui*, it is necessary to learn basic vocabulary. An understanding of the terms "auspicious and inauspicious," "*yin* and *yang*," as well as the composition of the five elements, is essential. The terms auspicious and inauspicious are commonly used in *feng shui* and mean "favorable" or "bringing good fortune" and "not favorable" or "bringing bad fortune." An arrangement that is auspicious is considered to be conducive to success, health, and prosperity. Inauspicious designs are considered unlucky, leading to unfortunate circumstances, discomfort, and even disease. Although this distinction creates a black-and-white view of what is good and bad, it is the mixture of different auspicious and inauspicious elements in the home that creates varying shades of gray.

Figure 6. *Yin-yang* symbol

The terms *yin* and *yang* are well known and the *yin-yang* symbol is easily recognized (Figure 6). The symbol represents balance and harmony, profound concepts with endless applications. *Yin* and *yang* are ancient Chinese terms that represent the complementary forces that form the universe. One force acts upon the other and, in their balance, harmony is achieved. *Yin* energy represents stillness, darkness, and attributes associated with death, while *yang* represents forces that create energy, movement, color, excitement, noise, and light. Excesses of either state will create disharmony. Environments with more *yang* energy will generate excitement. For example, while strolling down the strip in Las Vegas, one is subjected to bright, blinking lights and many sounds, which create energy and excitement everywhere. Contrast that to the quiet, bland solitude of a silent meditation room or a cemetery, which are environments dominated by the *yin* force.

In nature, both *yin* and *yang* are represented in everything, everywhere. This interplay needs to be manually created in the home. In general, we want our homes to be more *yang* than *yin*, with the exception of the adult bedrooms. Take a walk around your house and see if you can identify which rooms should be more *yin* or more *yang*.

The five elements

In *feng shui*, all materials are divided up into one of five categories, called elements. The elements in ancient Chinese tradition are earth, fire, water, wood, and metal. These are abstractions. For example, the wood element can be represented by a piece of wood, but also by a plant which can generate wood. The fire element can be represented by a light fixture or merely the color red. The different elements affect each other. For example, a fire element in the home can undo the energetic effect of a nearby wood element as fire burns wood for fuel.

The earth element is a force of stability. It represents the energy of natural harmony and is important to anchor the center of your home. Examples of a few "earthy" decorative materials include ceramics, crystals, and stones. Colors used to represent the earth element include beige, clay/mud colors, terra cotta, sandy tones, and even light yellows. Consider that new earth is created by fire, so in areas of the home that are earth-centered, it is important to place fire elements. Just as plants and trees consume the earth to grow, wood elements will weaken the earth-centered areas of your home. Similarly, metal is created by earth and therefore takes energy from the earth, so it is a good idea to reduce the presence of wood and metals in areas of your home that are designated for a strong earth energy.

The fire element is a powerful *yang* force associated with transformation, creation, and success. Both natural and artificial sources of light generate fire energy. Big windows will allow fire energy into a room. Candles and lamps can also create fire energy. Fire energy is most important in the southern rooms of your home. Vibrant reds, oranges, yellows, purples, and pinks emphasize the fire element. Since fire uses wood for fuel, it is important to place wood elements in rooms dominated by the fire element. A small water feature is a useful addition to a room with fire energy because the fire can symbolically turn the water into steam and generate power. Too large a water feature, however, can drown the fire and deplete the fire's power. Fire energy will destroy metal, so metal objects are not helpful in rooms with prevailing fire energy.

The water element is an extremely powerful force and needs to be controlled. Think of the power in a tsunami. Water energy is a *yin* force and is represented by darker colors such as blacks and blues. Water energy is most powerful when placed in the northern part of your home, or outside your home to the north. Plants can stimulate the water element, as can water features such as small indoor fountains. Because metals can turn into a liquid state, they simulate water and can be placed in areas of the home with a water dominance.

The wood element symbolizes growth and potential. As wood is burned by fire a room representing the fire element can have wood, but a room designated to promote the wood element should not have fire represented. Water features enhance the energy of wood since water helps plants to grow. Metals destroy wood and should be avoided in rooms that are designed to promote the wood energy. Wood is most effective when placed in the east and southeast parts of your home. In the home, wood can be symbolized by the placement of indoor plants that are alive, dried, or even artificial. It is the symbolism of the element that is most important. Browns and greens, like the colors of trees and woody plants, are optimal for representing the wood element.

Metal energy symbolizes wealth and can be represented by coins and other metallic materials. Although metal is symbolic of abundance, it is cold and devoid of life. There is a proper place in the home for metal, but it should be placed with material representing the earth element because metal is created from earth. An example of this would be placing metallic coins in a ceramic dish. Water should be avoided in the metal centers of your home because water weakens metal energy. Although the metal element is barren and lifeless, it helps create energetic movement within the home, important for good *feng shui*. Areas of the house emphasizing the metal element can be painted gray or white. Metal energy can be emphasized by placing a jar of coins or decorative metallic objects in the appropriate rooms, typically the west and northwest rooms of the home.

Compass work

Everything in the home relates to everything else, and each element has auspicious locations within the home, based on compass direction. It is therefore necessary to know how your home sits in the world and which direction your home faces. *Feng shui* practitioners utilize a compass to determine a building's location and design. Land formations such as hills and valleys, water elements such as streams, rivers, and ponds, and vegetation are all considered when determining the optimal placement for a new home. In general, the home's back should be protected by a hill or tall trees, while the front should be wide open and inviting. Water, or in our modern world, a street, should be within view and gently flowing toward the front of the house. Even if a home is not ideally placed, design of the home's interior can optimize energy flow within and around the home.

The first step of compass work is to draw a scaled diagram of your home's main floor. This is most easily accomplished on grid paper. All parts of the home should be included. A home's shape may be a simple square, a rectangle, or an oblong shape with extensions. Next, use a compass to superimpose the four cardinal directions: north, east, west, and south. Most smart phones have a preloaded compass app.

After creating an overall layout of the main floor, make layouts of each additional floor, demarcating bedrooms, the kitchen, bathrooms, living room, dining room, etc. The front entranceway should be clearly marked, for this is the most important passageway for energy to enter the home. Determine which direction the front door faces by standing inside the doorway with a compass and assessing its orientation. Then, note this direction on the diagram.

Create a grid of nine squares or rectangles for each layout by dividing the length and width into three equal segments. If the home has extensions, some *feng shui* practitioners will draw a separate grid for each one. Once the grids are created, place a compass in the center of the middle square, and draw lines emanating from the center outward toward the eight compass directions. Then, orient the perimeter of the house into eight quadrants: north, northeast, east, southeast, south, etc. The center of the home is also marked. My home diagram ended up looking like that shown in Figure 7.

Figure 7. A sample home compass drawing - main floor

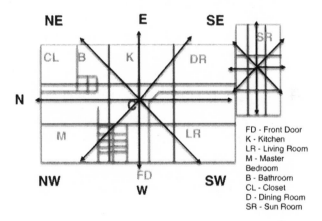

The ancient Chinese *Lo Shu* square will help you organize the energy flow throughout your home (Figure 8). In this diagram, the sum of each three-digit line, whether horizontal, vertical, or diagonal, adds up to fifteen, indicating the numbers are placed in perfect balance.

Figure 8. *Lo Shu* square

4	9	2
3	5	7
8	1	6

Each section of the home, regardless of its utilitarian function, is located in a part of the house designated to receive energy from a specific element. Rooms that face north are important for career advancement and should emphasize the water element. The northeast corner of the home generates spiritual growth and should emphasize the earth element. The east room is the seat of health and should bring out the wood element. The southeastern quadrant of the home is the source for abundance, and will strengthen with the wood element. Rooms to the south house one's reputation, receiving power through the fire element. The southwest quadrant is the area for love and will strengthen by emphasizing the earth element. Creativity is generated in the west, which should feature the metal element. Finally, the northwest is a home's link to community and the appreciation for others. This quadrant should be enhanced by energy from the metal element. The center of the home is grounded by the earth element. The resulting energy reference guide is referred to as a *Bagua* map (Figure 9).

Figure 9: *Bagua* Map

NW Metal Appreciation for others	N Water Career advancement	NE Earth Spiritual development
W Creativity Metal	Center Earth Grounding	E Wood Health
SW Earth Love	S Fire Reputation	SE Wood Abundance

The process

Overlay a *Bagua* map onto each floor plan. In order to get used to the element represented in each room of the house, write the element name on a sticky note and place it on the corresponding wall in each room to give a little reminder each time the room is entered. Now, it is time to disassemble and rework each room, one at a time.

Before any rearrangement, first energize the corner of each room by placing something in the corner of the corresponding direction that emphasizes the room's element. For example, in the above diagram, because the master bedroom (M) faces north, the water element should dominate, so a dark blue decorative item should be placed in the northern corner of the room. Red painted pottery in the southern corner of the sun room will emphasize the fire element.

After energizing each room, begin reducing clutter. Too much stuff, whether it's on your countertops, in your closet, or under your bed, can cause energy stagnation. A home needs active movement of *chi* and not the stagnation that results from an accumulation of items from the past. Energy stagnation and confusion can negatively affect many areas of your life. By decluttering, you'll create room for *chi* to bring new opportunities into your home and to you. This is an essential step in the creation of a harmonious house.

Rid yourself of items that make you, or anyone else who shares the space, feel shame, guilt, remorse, sadness, anger, or resentment. If an object causes negative emotion, dispose of it. If an object ties you to the past, prohibiting you from being present in your daily life, dispose of it. As you evaluate each object, reflect on what it represents for you. When did you get it? Was it a happy time or a difficult time? Did someone give the item to you as a gift? Is that person still in your life? Do you love having it and seeing it? Or does the object create guilt, remorse, or a sense of missed opportunity?

If you share a room with another, such as a master bedroom, the energy needs to be agreeable to both of you. If an object makes either one of you feel bad because it represents a part of an older life or older relationship that is no longer relevant, it should be discarded. In a family room, everyone in the family should feel comfortable. If a displayed item makes anyone in the family unhappy, it should be removed. For example, if only one child won a trophy at an event where other children competed, displaying the winner's trophy in the family room may cause the other children to feel bad. It is better to have your children put trophies in their own bedrooms or any other special place that is "theirs." In this way, every member of your household will feel comfortable and welcome in every room of the house.

In *feng shui*, your whole house, including the storage areas, are a representation of you. So, cleaning house doesn't mean throw in everything you don't want or need into the attic and closet. Closets need to be decluttered too. If closets are filled with items that you haven't thought about or looked at for over five years, sell them, donate them, or throw them away. This process will lighten up your home. Clean out the refrigerator and straighten out kitchen cabinets, drawers, and storage areas. After decluttering a room or closet, avoid re-accumulating clutter there in the future.

After cleanup, consider each room's function and determine if the room should be more *yin* or *yang* energy. Bedrooms, meditation rooms, and places where one desires peace and quiet need to be more *yin*. Soft lighting, muted colors, and comfortable surroundings are examples of *yin* decor. Stressful images, blinking lights, electronic equipment, exercise equipment, bright colors, and so on should not be placed in a *yin* environment, especially in an adult's bedroom. Communal rooms, such as the kitchen, living room, dining room, playroom, and entertainment room should all emphasize stronger *yang* energy. Children's bedrooms should also emphasize *yang*, which will provide energy for growth and development. Decorate these rooms with brighter colors and dynamic pieces of artwork. Electronic equipment, such as televisions, music systems, and computers contribute to *yang* energy. By reflecting energy, mirrors are effective in *yang*-oriented rooms. The dining room is an excellent place to hang a big mirror for it will reflect the abundance of food served at each meal.

After this ground work, it is time to work on each room layout and more specific design concepts. In designing each room, the most important initial consideration is the movement of *chi* into and throughout the room. Imagine *chi* as a river of energy that comes into the room through the door. When that energy hits a piece of furniture, it washes right and left of the object, and continues its movement. When the energy encounters a second door or a window, it flows out of the room and potentially out of the house. The goal in designing each room layout is to have the *chi* swirl through and fill the room, touching each of the pieces of furniture before exiting. Energy flow can be manipulated by the placement of both furniture and decorative objects.

Two additional concepts for consideration when designing each room are poison arrows and symbols. Poison arrows create negative *chi.* They are generated by anything that cuts or pierces the energy in a room. Protruding corners from furniture and window ledges are common sources of poison arrows. Additional examples include spiky plants such as cacti and open book shelves, which can slice the energy in a room. The lines created by these shapes cut the air in front of the object. If you are in the path of the arrow, it can pierce your energy, causing you a negative energy flow.

Masking or "treating" a poison arrow is achieved by applying a structure that will symbolically diffuse the hardness or sharpness of the arrow, called a deflector. A piece of fabric, a plant, a hanging crystal or wind chime, or any other decorative element can be placed in front of a poison arrow to dissipate its potency. If the object deflects your attention away from the corner, then it works. It's really as simple as that. You can use anything you'd like to deflect a poison arrow except for another poison arrow.

Symbolism, an important part of the *feng shui* practice, is found in all cultures. A symbol is a physical representation of a mood, thought, or idea. Symbols create a vibe or energy when looked at. We are surrounded by symbols at home and in our public spaces, each of which can have different meanings depending on one's perspective. A symbol can take on different meanings depending on the sound it makes, the smell it emanates, and its color. For example, the heart shape is a symbol of love. A red heart has a different connotation, however, than a blue heart. Although subtle, the placement of symbols can manipulate the moods and disposition of the people in a living space.

As you design each room, decorative objects, paint colors, and flooring choices should mostly conform to the element represented in each room. So, in rooms that face the northwest, the water element should determine the choice of colors: blues, blacks, and greens. Place metallic items in the northwest. Contrast this to the south-facing room, which houses the fire element and should contain red tones, deep pinks, and oranges with some blues to represent the water element. The earth-centered rooms would have items that represent earth energy, such as pieces of pottery, shells, rocks, and crystals with color schemes such as browns, beiges, and other earthy tones. Place symbols in each room to focus energy and to bring you abundance, love, and joy. Many online guides are available to provide ideas of how to emphasize the different elements. Be creative and playful. Have fun and be lighthearted as you take time to decorate.

Specific rooms: the entranceway

The most important space in your home is the front door and entranceway. The front door is the symbolic mouth of your home through which *chi* enters. If access to the front door is inviting and wide open, a sufficient amount of *chi* can enter. However, if the entryway is obstructed by structures or overgrown shrubs, the amount of *chi* entering the home will be deficient. Therefore, the orientation and width of your front walkway are important, as are the size and location of shrubs and trees that greet visitors as they walk to your door. Placing a front door behind a hill or blockade of some sort is certainly inauspicious.

Making an entryway beautiful will improve the quality of *chi* that circulates throughout your house. Remove any non-decorative items by your front door, such as children's toys, bicycles, garbage bins, chipped pots, etc. Trim overgrown shrubs and low branches crowding the walkway to your door. Keep the walkway swept clean. If the door squeaks when opened, spray the hinges with lubricant. Paint the front door a color that is harmonious with the element corresponding to the door's direction. The front door should be noticed and should not blend in with the rest of the house.

Bedrooms

A bedroom with good *feng shui* will provide the occupant with comfort and protection during sleep and a safe haven for romance and lovemaking. There are special considerations for the adult bedroom that allow the proper flow of *chi*. First, the bed should not be placed on a wall directly in front of the doorway, but rather on an opposing wall, caddy- corner to the door. If the bed is placed directly in front of the doorway, it will be bombarded with too much *chi*, creating unrest in the bed. If there is no alternative, a screen or a piece of furniture can be placed between the bed and the door to deflect the *chi*. A bed should not be placed directly beneath a window, for this arrangement will allow the *chi* to pass over the bed and out the window, creating insecurity. Placing a bed underneath a slanted ceiling is also inauspicious. This arrangement causes constriction of the energy flow to the bed and can create emotional instability and lower energy levels in the bed's occupants. The bed should be high enough off the ground so that *chi* can flow beneath it. The underside of the bed should not be used for storage as this will block the flow of *chi*. Once the bed is properly placed, pieces of furniture should be placed on either side of the bed to create a setting, grounding the bed.

An adult bedroom should emphasize *yin* energy and so *feng shui* masters recommend doing away with all *yang* elements in the bedroom, including mirrors. If a mirror needs to be placed in a bedroom, it should not face or reflect the bed. This is particularly important for a couple as the reflection of the couple in bed subtly suggests the introduction of additional beings, which can eventually destroy the relationship. Other *yang* elements, including office work, exercise equipment, and electronics, should not be placed in the bedroom, but rather in a part of the house that is more *yang* oriented. Placing a TV and related electronics within a cabinet that can be closed for concealment may be an acceptable alternative for some.

After placing bedroom furniture, search for poison arrows pointing toward the bed. As you discover each one, create a deflector. Finally, place symbols in the bedroom to encourage harmony, success, and joy for you and your partner. These personal items will help to maintain a strong relationship between the two of you.

A child's bed should be placed utilizing similar concepts as described for the adult bed. A child's bedroom, however, should emphasize *yang* energy. It is okay to have a mirror and electronic gadgets in a child's bedroom. In addition, posters and artwork should display more vibrant, energetic scenes.

Kitchen

The kitchen is a laboratory where fire or heating elements are used to create a meal from foods. Ideally, the kitchen should be located in a part of the house that suffers from *chi* deficiency. Placement of the oven and range are particularly important, for these units significantly enhance *chi*. The oven should not be placed in line with the front door of the house and mirrors should not be placed to reflect the oven or range. Both of these arrangements can create too much of the fire element and be a set-up for possible fire from excessive *chi*. On the other hand, the oven and range should also not be placed adjacent to the sink, as the water element can squelch the fire production.

Family room

The family room is the place where everyone should be able to relax without the worry of breaking or destroying things. The most comfortable family rooms have casual furniture, including footrests. The flooring should also be cozy and comfortable. Family accomplishments and pictures of relatives and friends should be displayed. The family room is the best location for electronics and for playing games.

Feng shui – an ongoing process

After completing a room, take a few deep breaths, clear your mind, and walk back into each room that you have worked on and take note of how you feel upon entering. Is the room welcoming? Relaxing? Peaceful? Are you happy with it? If not, make some changes and see how those changes work for you. *Feng shui* is a dynamic process that actually becomes a way of life. These concepts can be applied to as many rooms in the home as desired. It is impossible to get a home to be 100% concordant with the rules of *feng shui*, but each step made in that direction will bring dwellers a greater sense of harmony, which will influence their endeavors outside the home.

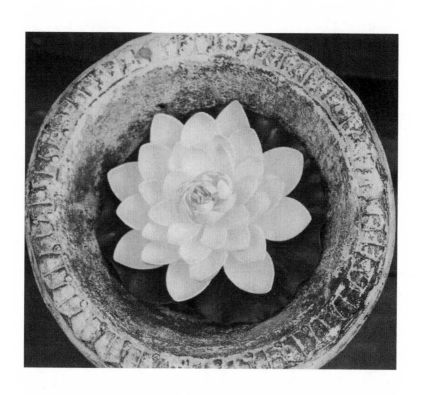

Chapter 12

MEDITATION

A person's thought process and state of consciousness can perhaps be the most toxic element in the home. In order to understand how our thoughts affect our well-being, it is necessary to become introspective and do work within.

Most of us run around daily, living on automatic pilot. Rituals and obligations, such as going to work, taking care of children, doing laundry, going shopping, and maintaining the home occupy most days. Most tasks become routinized and mindless. However, problems and adversity are a common occurrence and depending on one's personality, negative thoughts from these experiences may hang on. Over time, these fragments of hurt, irritation, and annoyance build up, affecting us emotionally and spiritually. Our minds play reruns over and over again, causing emotional suffering. Memories may fade, but displaced anger, depression, lethargy, or confusion may persist.

Physical disease can result from an unhealthy mind. The definition of somatization is the manifestation of symptoms in the body created by the mind. Physical diseases often occur from forms of chronic stress. Life is richly layered with undercurrents, most of which we are not aware of on a conscious level. Whether or not sources of stress relate to tasteless contaminants in the air, food, water, unseen currents of energy moving through the home, or emotional baggage, these elements all affect one's well-being.

Dreams provide clues to the problems and puzzles the mind is currently trying to resolve. Dream interpretation is an extremely helpful tool to clean out the debris from the subconscious mind. Jungian analysis is a form of psychotherapy that explores the realm of dreams. By interpreting the psyche's use of symbols represented by various scenes, people, and objects, this analysis is able to uncover the interplay of the subconscious emotions and conflicts we experience in our day-to-day life. Through dream analysis, we can dissolve the buildup of psychological stress that can cause us to stall emotionally and perhaps deteriorate physically.

It has been said over and over again by counselors, life coaches, sports coaches, and spiritual leaders that "attitude is everything." With regard to creating a conscious home, one's mind needs to be in the right place. Otherwise, it doesn't matter how well the rest of the home is fixed up. This chapter is last, because it will require the most work. Unlike the one-time purchase of a water purifier or perhaps watering houseplants a few times a week, meditation requires daily effort. You may be thinking that you don't have any more time in the day to give up for meditation, but it will need to become a priority.

I recently had a conversation with a colleague about our lifestyles. He was stressed. He complained that working a full-time job and helping to take care of his children left him with no free time for himself. Every moment that he was away from work, he felt he needed to be doing something for his wife or his children. I listened to him, knowing that he was blessed to be in a career that afforded him a lot of time off, much more than most others who work for a living. Yet, despite all of this time off, he still felt overwhelmed, rushing to get things done. Time management is crucial.

"Not enough time" is a sentiment most people can resonate with. With constant distraction and interruptions during the day, time erodes away. The number of times a typical person in today's world checks their cell phone for a message, call, email, or app notification is astounding. Keeping up with never-ending correspondence is a major source of stress, for we are absorbed in a virtual world where we are never caught up, never able to sit back and relax for any extended period of time.

Before the Internet, which wasn't that long ago, there was no email or text messaging. There were no smartphones. The older members of our society remember a time when there were no answering machines or caller ID boxes. If you weren't home, you had no idea if someone had tried to call you. When you talked to someone on the phone, you were forced to stay in one room, for there were no portable phones, so you might have sprawled on the couch or on the floor with your feet up on the wall while talking to your friend or to family, and it was fun. Calling someone "long distance" meant that you had to pay extra money for each minute that you talked to someone on the phone, so we wrote and read letters. Life was much more relaxed. Contrast that with today, where people commonly check messages and emails even when they are dining out in an expensive restaurant. Today, you have to create and preserve free time.

Now, I do admit, carrying the world's collective brain on my phone is awesome. But I try to control my use by carving out a finite amount of time for correspondence and information review each day, rather than responding to every beep and ringtone like one of Pavlov's dogs. Many parents set time limits for how long their children can stay on their devices each day. The truth is that we should all set limits in order to open up free time for ourselves.

Budgeting time is crucial. Even retired people can find that their schedules are completely filled up and may feel stressed out because they are too busy. Budget time as if it were currency. And when you do, allot at least thirty minutes a day for yourself. Time without your children, spouse, friends, or work. This is not a time for cleaning, going through the mail, making phone calls, watching TV, reading, or playing on a device. This time, without any work, social interaction, or passive entertainment of any kind, should be spent in contemplation through meditation.

If you were to research the beneficial health effects attributed to the daily practice of meditation, you might be motivated to start the practice today. Thousands of peer-reviewed publications in medical journals have documented positive health effects from meditation, even at only twenty minutes a day. Decreased rates of heart disease and depression, lower blood pressure and pulse rates, and decreased stress have been observed with people who practice meditation.[1] The beneficial effects of meditation also include strengthening of the immune system, reducing inflammation, and improving the immune response,[2] which are extraordinarily important for good health. People who practice daily meditation effectively can sometimes decrease or even stop taking medications. Daily meditation has even been characterized as being healthier than exercise.[3]

Meditation has been credited with causing cellular as well as genetic effects, including the reduction of cellular aging.[4] That means that nuclei of individual cells in the body change which proteins they make when you meditate, which in turn, changes your physiology. Think about that for a moment. The mind can control the behavior of individual cells in the body! Meditation improves your physical and mental health by helping to prevent multiple diseases, making you happier, and improving the abilities of both your body and mind.

Making the daily commitment to let go of a piece of your busy life, both by taking the time and also by relaxing your mind, is perhaps the hardest part of the discipline. You can purchase books about meditation, listen to audio files to help guide you through meditation, or even pay for meditation classes. But you have to allot the time and provide the mental clarity in your busy day for this process.

Before reserving a block of time to meditate each day, decide on how you want to spend the time. Thousands of meditation techniques exist, varying from active forms such as yoga or *tai chi*, to sitting still in a lotus position. Consider whether you initially want to do an active discipline, such as yoga, or a static form, such as focusing on a candle flame while clearing the mind, or focusing on a single thought or mantra. Consider the technique as a vehicle to move you down the path to awareness and consciousness. All meditation techniques can be effective—think of them as paths that lead to the same place.

Logistics will differ. For example, if you are going to attend an organized class, you will need to arrange your schedule around the class meeting time. If you opt for a solitary form of meditation, you will have greater flexibility in carving out a time slot that suits your needs, but you will need a room or place to go without distractions. A combination of techniques can also be productive. After a little bit of research and thought, look at your weekly schedule and figure out when you can set this time each day.

Mindfulness meditation

The easiest entrée to meditation is to learn how to become present and live in "the now." The term given to this state of being is "mindfulness." This discipline has been shown scientifically to have profound positive health effects for those who practice it. Mindfulness requires detaching from your emotions, or reflexive personality, and becoming more self- aware. This is a great way for a novice to enter into the realm of meditation and to gain health benefits quickly.

The simplest method to start becoming mindful is to focus on the breath. This can be done while sitting on a meditation pillow, resting in bed, or while walking down the street. The practice of mindfulness trains the mind to dismiss distractions. If practiced regularly, this exercise will have a profound effect on reducing baseline stress levels.

Before starting meditation, decide on which way you would like to gauge time. Would you prefer to count your heart beats or to count seconds in your mind? Either will work well, but don't watch a clock, for that will prevent full entrainment. I prefer to count heart beats and will describe the process with that method. Don't be concerned about accuracy. Just go with what you think is right. No pressure. No worries.

Begin by taking in a slow, deep breath through your nose and as you do, become aware of your breath. As you inhale, either count to three seconds in your mind, or sense your heart beat and count three heart beats. Become aware of the feeling of your chest expanding and of your diaphragm pressing down. Hold your breath for three beats while you feel the satisfaction of having your lungs filled with nourishing air. Then exhale, letting your breath out through your mouth, again counting three beats in your mind. Focus on your breath exiting out of your mouth and feel your chest and diaphragm relax. Do this breathing cycle one more time. Then, repeat the process with a four-beat count for each step. Take another deep, satisfying four-beat breath and, again, concentrate on the rush of air as it moves into and fills your lungs. Feel your chest expand and again, hold that breath for four beats. Then, relax and be aware as the breath leaves your chest over a four-beat interval.

This regulated breath is simple to do and yet very effective. As you initially perform this series of controlled breaths, it should be easy to concentrate on the technique. Your pulse will slow as your heart beat entrains with your breath. Your mind will follow by slowing down its frenzy. But after a few cycles, your mind will more than likely start to wander off. That's okay. Become aware of the thoughts that come into your mind and then let each of them go, without attachment, as if they were flowing away down a stream. You are becoming "present." You will become less aware of your physical body and its sensations in this state of consciousness. Maintain this breath control, preferably for twenty minutes or so. Even touching the surface of this mind state for only three minutes while waiting in line in a market is beneficial. When you "wake up" from this focus, you will feel refreshed. This is a healthy way to take a quick break during a hectic day.

Yoga

Yoga is a grouping of ancient disciplines that predate Hinduism and have been dated back to 1700 BC. In fact, some yoga masters consider the discipline to be over 40,000 years old! The word yoga means "union," a perfect word to describe the goal of these disciplines, which is to access and strengthen the bridge between an individual's consciousness and the collective or universal consciousness.

Yoga uses a triad of physical posturing, breath control, and meditation to achieve this union. These techniques are integrated to achieve a balance of the mind, body, and spirit. Posturing brings one's conscious awareness to the physical body. Qualities such as strength versus weakness and rigidity versus flexibility are tested, observed, and developed, with the goal of developing a balance between strength and flexibility.

The cyclic, rhythmic nature of the breath is considered to be the life force, representing a link between the physical and the spiritual. The meditative component allows one to detach the mind from the body in order to strengthen connection to the spiritual realm.

Yoga creates a sense of peace and well-being. As the practitioner develops technique to go deeper into focus, he/she will begin to feel harmony with and diminished aggression toward the surrounding environment and other beings in their world.[5] Like all forms of meditation, yoga will bring about emotional stability and increased clarity of mind.[6]

Yoga is multifaceted, consisting of eight different limbs or branches, each emphasizing different aspects of the discipline. Depending on one's philosophy, spiritual beliefs, and needs, one or another form of yoga may be chosen for practice. In the US, the most common form of yoga is referred to as hatha yoga, or the yoga of postures. There are many different styles within this branch, but each incorporates postures with breath control and meditation. Yoga should be taught by an instructor, someone with sufficient experience who can guide the student through the discipline. Books written about yoga technique can also be helpful. Incorporate yoga into daily life in order to gain the discipline's benefits. By doing so, the body and mind will become strong, pliant, flexible, and healthy.

Qi gong and *tai chi*

Qi gong is a group of ancient Chinese disciplines that, similar to yoga, integrate the mind, body, and spirit. Qi, pronounced "chi", is the same energy flow manipulated in *feng shui*. The name *qi gong* literally means "cultivating energy." By performing these disciplines, vital energy is produced, which can then be used to heal oneself from injuries and illness. *Qi gong* will increase the practitioner's overall wellness and rejuvenate the mind and body. There are many documented, positive health effects attributed to the daily practice of both *qi gong* and *tai chi*, involving most of the organ systems, including the immune system.[7]

Some styles of *qi gong* require movement, while others are based on stationary posturing, similar to yoga. Movement may be slow and flowing as with *tai chi*, or rapid and deliberate as with kung fu. Some forms of *qi gong* are more appropriate for the elderly, while others would be more beneficial for children. The style of discipline that resonates with one's needs and personality should be chosen. More competitive and aggressive people may find a form of kung fu to be more suitable, whereas non- confrontational individuals may enjoy learning and practicing *tai chi*.

Tai chi is an ancient form of *qi gong* that incorporates meditation with slow, focused movement and controlled breath. This discipline will generate and circulate one's internal energy. During *tai chi* work, the body is in constant motion. As with yoga, not all forms of *tai chi* are alike. Each style of *tai chi* emphasizes a different aspect of the discipline. Some schools are more geared toward optimizing health, while others are focused on the martial art and closer to a style of kung fu. After learning how to perform these movements under the guidance of an instructor, these exercises can be practiced anywhere, alone or with a group. Given the motion and more dynamic nature of this discipline, it may be more appealing to some than yoga. *Tai chi*, or any form of *qi gong*, will help one create and maintain a healthy mind, based on harmony, stability, and joy. It is an excellent discipline to help one "detox" from life's daily stressors.

Transcendental meditation

Transcendental meditation (TM), the first meditation technique introduced to Western cultures in the 1960s, introduced Westerners to the concept of the "unified field" through meditation.[8] Other terms given to the unified field include the collective consciousness, mind of God, and quantum field. TM became a popular method to become spiritually "in tuned," or enlightened, without becoming a monk, or converting to Krishnaism or Buddhism. It certainly helped that the Beatles, Mick Jagger, Donovan, and other celebrities studied TM with the Maharishi Yogi in India, and brought TM to the mainstream pop culture.

Many studies in peer-reviewed literature document the health benefits of TM. The daily practice of TM can improve some mood disorders by reducing stress and preventing and managing anxiety, which are the cause of many diseases and disorders in our culture. TM has been helpful in treating insomnia and increasing clarity of thought. Measurable effects from the daily practice of TM include documented reduction in atherosclerosis plaque burden, lowering blood pressure, increasing longevity, and others.[9] TM is a meditation technique taught by certified TM instructors and requires an ongoing investment in order to remain in training. Although costly, it can be tremendously helpful to have a meditation teacher and/ or a coach to help keep you accountable to the discipline. TM requires an investment of twenty minutes, twice a day, to achieve its results. Although I have not personally studied TM, I do have several good friends who studied TM for years and found the discipline to be very valuable. Although the world of meditation is ultimately limitless and independent of any one method or organization, TM is a well-researched and organized group which an initiate may want to investigate.

Walking meditation

Walking meditation is a very traditional method of meditation you can use to become grounded and to connect with your spirit. There are several ways to practice this form of meditation, each requiring the controlled focus of your mind. It is ideal to pick a place to walk where you are not going to run into people you know or who will otherwise distract you. Ideally, you would walk on a path or in a yard, alone.

In one method, you walk at a slow pace and, while breathing in and out deeply, place your focus on your feet as you take each step. You can feel the pressure on your toes as you lift off your foot. Feel the ground as you then place your foot down and shift your weight. After several steps, you can move your consciousness outside of your body to become aware of the ground that you are stepping on. With each step, you are shifting grains of soil, sand, or pebbles. Or perhaps you are crumpling grass or snapping small twigs with each step. Become aware of how you are changing the earth by walking on it. As extraneous thoughts pop up into your mind, acknowledge them and then let them go. Try to clear your mind and refocus on your feet and start the process over again. Even after ten minutes, you will feel rejuvenated and refreshed.

An alternative method of walking meditation is to completely detach your conscious mind from your physical body and its sensations and to focus instead on the horizon. While staring at the horizon, go into a trance, and then bring into your mind a singular thought. Perhaps you are looking for joy in your life. Focus on the horizon and imagine the word "joy" is written there for you to observe. Say and repeat the word quietly to yourself slowly as you walk forward. If you prefer, a symbol can be substituted for a word. A short phrase, such as a mantra, can also be visualized and repeated softly to yourself while engaged in walking meditation. When the words dissipate, stop walking. Close your eyes for a moment. Reopen them and refocus on the horizon. Bring up the image you would like to manifest and begin walking again, maintaining your focus for as long as you can. Repeat the process each time you lose focus.

There are no restrictions to what you can visualize during this discipline, but it is important to distance yourself from any emotional reactions to your image or words. In addition, the goal with walking meditation is to achieve a deepened state of meditative focus rather than walking a great distance. In fact, you may not actually walk very far at all. The intensity of the focus is what matters.

Candle meditation

Candle meditation is my personal favorite. When I was taught to meditate by using a candle flame, I was instructed to focus on the dark part of the flame and to "go there." As with all forms of meditation, it is necessary to pick a time of day when there are not going to be any foreseeable interruptions. Make sure the ringer on your home phone is turned off and that your cell phone is placed in airplane mode.

Soft, instrumental music can be played in the background, music that will entrain you and will bring you into a relaxed state. Avoid music with lyrics for the words can be distracting, and they can corrupt the process by putting the lyricist's thoughts into your mind during your meditative focus. Light a small beeswax or soy candle and draw the curtains to darken the room so that the only light in the room is emanating from the candle flame. Be careful to place the candle in a secure holder. Finally, sit cross- legged in a lotus position on a small pillow to raise your butt up off of the ground.

Be totally still while gazing into the center of the candle flame. Initially, focusing on the breath will help to relax and calm the mind. As breathing becomes more regular, little thoughts may start to pop up into your mind. Acknowledge them and let them dissipate. As you become conscious and detached from your thoughts, you reach a deep state of relaxation. In this state, you can now place a symbol, a word, or a mantra into the candle flame, much like you do with the walking meditation. Don't think about the impact of the words or how they make you feel. Just observe them. If you lose focus, bring your attention back to the breath and begin the process again. With practice, this powerful discipline will bring you to very deep levels of meditative focus.

As mentioned earlier, it doesn't really matter which form of meditation you choose to study, for all of these disciplines will provide a chance for your mind to unwind and recharge and time for your body to heal.

A giant leap into the unknown

The meditative state is a powerful place to work from. Yes, there is scientific proof that this state of mind can lower one's baseline stress response and help the body heal. But the effects of meditation go beyond the psychological and physiological. As one becomes more adept at meditation, it becomes clearer that there are many levels of consciousness to explore, not simply the conscious state and the meditative state. The deeper the level you go down to, the more profound the effects your meditation may have.

It has been suggested that meditation connects one to the collective consciousness, a timeless realm. By connecting to this state, meditation can be used to create a future experience, a new attitude, or even a new relationship. In this space, one may also "download" information that "pops up" into your head; some refer to this as having a "stroke of genius." This is precisely the method with which many scientists and artists have generated their most impactful work. You may have read that Paul McCartney "woke up" and wrote down the music to his extraordinarily impactful song *Yesterday*. It was already written and the music was already composed in his head. All he had to do was write the words and music down when he came around.

One of Albert Einstein's more famous quotes acknowledges this process:

> The intellect has little to do on the road to discovery. There comes a leap in consciousness, call it intuition or what you will, and the solution comes to you, and you don't know how or why.

Getting access to this state can happen in the blink of an eye, but it can also take years of practice. The rapidity depends on one's intensity of focus. The process cannot be rushed and you cannot "will" it to happen with your personality. Meditation requires being in a trance-like state. Sitting in a dark room with the candle lit and "thinking" is not going to bring you into an altered state.

The ability of some people to focus on "an intention" is one of the characteristics that allows them to enjoy great success in their life. Certainly, some people have this innate ability, while others are mired in confusion and chaos, constantly struggling to maintain a disciplined mind. Chaos has its place, but it is vitally important to be able to focus on an intention and to "create reality." If you are one who is usually confused, running around in circles trying to get things done, you are not alone. But it would behoove you to start training your mind to become more focused. Maintaining focused attention is a skill that improves with practice. After periods of meditation, you may find that you are filled with ideas. Write them down! Make a list and get organized for the time in between meditation sessions. This will help you experience your life in a more productive way in between your brief sessions of "creating" your life. This will sound mysterious to some, ridiculous to others, and yet will ring true to many. Understanding this as truth will only happen after you gain the wisdom from repeated experience for yourself. You will eventually come to appreciate that:

What You Think About Each Day Matters

It's a quick blip of a statement, yet it has profound implications. It is true, our thoughts make a difference, not only in the way we see the world and interpret our surroundings, but our thoughts can effect change by themselves. How you perceive a situation or what you think about another person can have a profound effect on both. It is not just that thinking positive is better than thinking negative; it goes way beyond that. Our thoughts and expectations shape our future reality. In fact, it has been suggested that we create our reality all of the time with every thought and decision we make throughout the day. Even transient thoughts during the day influence your world. The power of intention is significantly stronger, however, when one's mind is focused and free of distraction. Many spiritual teachers have taught this lesson.

One thing I have learned over the years is that the brain does not understand negatives. So, if you focus on not wanting something, you are actually putting your mind on the very thing that you don't want to happen and it will likely manifest as if you did want it to happen. One will experience a different kind of life by focusing on wants instead of things not wanted. Both modes of thought will manifest, but with different outcomes.

The ability to manifest isn't limited to adults. In fact, I've noticed that children are actually more adept at manifestation than adults. Perhaps this is because children's minds are less cluttered. Imagine teaching your child how to ride a bicycle. If the child is afraid of falling and sees one small rock in the middle of a wide road, the child will fear running over the rock and falling. Next thing you know, the child has indeed fallen off the bicycle and is lying right next to the rock screaming, "I knew I was going to fall on that rock!" Then, the blame comes.

It was, of course, the child's parent's fault that they didn't take the pebble off of the street. Another child who looks at the world as a source of limitless possibility would see a hundred other pathways to travel and never even come close to the stone.

We, as adults, aren't much different. It is hard to be in a relationship with someone who is always focusing on gloom and doom, or the potential negative side of outcomes, whether it's your child, spouse, or partner. It is impossible to sequester ourselves from naysayers. But we can protect ourselves by being that much more diligent in our commitments to focus and create wonderful opportunities, abundance, and joy. We can also teach those close to us that their thoughts matter too.

Active fears and phobias will also manifest. Many years ago, a close friend was terribly afraid of snakes and had a fear of snakes getting into her house. I had heard of snakes "appearing" in people's houses before, but I had never actually known anyone whom this had happened to personally. Her house was situated in front of dense woods, and although none of her neighbors had ever witnessed a snake in their houses, she was conscious of the possibility that a snake would enter her home. Sure enough, I received a call from her one afternoon and she told me there was a snake coiled up on the floor in her hallway! She didn't know how the snake had gotten into the home and so she continued to fear that another snake would enter her house. Several weeks later, another snake entered her house! After the second time, instead of remaining fearful, she altered her thought process. Although she still didn't know how the snakes had gotten into the home, she became proactive and cleaned up her yard and did what else she thought she needed to do to eliminate the snakes. Most importantly, her fear was gone. She hasn't had a problem since.

More examples of manifestation: some good, some bad.

In medicine, most physicians specialize, yet specialization comes at a mysterious potential cost. I have noticed a correlation between what a physician sub-specializes in and what they become afflicted with. A breast imager or breast surgeon will be more likely to develop breast cancer or have a wife with breast cancer than a physician specializing in orthopedics. A nephrologist (kidney doctor) may end up on dialysis or succumb to kidney or bladder cancer.

One of the most ridiculously blatant manifestations I experienced early on in my career was during my fellowship in orthopedic radiology. My team and I were studying the MRI appearance of wrist ligaments. We had created ligament tears in cadaveric wrists and then put them in an MRI scanner to see what they looked like. Although the MRI appearance of this type of injury hadn't been fully documented in the literature, it was well known at the time that wrist ligament tears were commonly caused by falling on an outstretched hand, known as a FOOSH injury. One night, during a break in my research, I ran out to get a quick dinner "to go." After getting my food, I walked through the restaurant quickly and exited the door. The sun was low in the sky and the light was flat. I began walking down the sidewalk, but soon tripped on a cement disc that had been left on the walkway where an umbrella had stood earlier in the day. My dinner went flying and I landed on both outstretched hands. And yes, I tore ligaments in both wrists. At the time, I considered this to be a bizarre coincidence. Now, I understand that this was a manifestation. I had spent many months focused on ligament tears and falling on outstretched hands, and so I brought it into my reality and experienced it for myself. Perhaps you've had a similar experience?

Knowing that many of us, particularly in the health profession, spend our days focusing on treating people who are sick or injured, it is important to spend time each day to "heal" ourselves. After finishing the day's tasks, it is helpful to meditate for a few moments to focus on perfect health, youthful energy, and unconditional love. It is also wonderful to start each day with meditation. Clearing the mind and then walking through the day in advance, detailing how things should unfold, can have a dramatic effect. Not every detail needs to be described, but stating with the affirmation every morning that you are feeling wonderful and healthy is a great start. You can start each day with the intentions that you are going to be filled with joy, achieve success in whatever you do, and that you will meet new, interesting people. Wouldn't that be a great way to spend the day? Give it a try. You might be surprised at how well your future days unfold.

About the Author

Rob Brown, MD, is a diagnostic radiologist who has worked in private practice and at academic centers, including NYU Medical Center and the Cleveland Clinic Foundation. He has helped train residents and medical students and written many journal articles in peer-reviewed publications and book chapters during his twenty-five-year career. His varied life experiences, including surviving cancer, have helped him understand how to best achieve wellness.

References

Introduction

1. Van Oostrom, S.H., et al. "Time Trends in Prevalence of Chronic Diseases and Multimorbidity not only Due to Aging: Data from General Practices and Health Surveys." *PLOS ONE*, August 2, 2016. doi: 10.1371/journal.pone.0160264.
2. Murray, C.J., Lopez, A.D. eds. "The Global Burden of Disease: A Comprehensive Assessment of Mortality and Disability from Diseases, Injuries, and Risk Factors in 1990 and Projected to 2020." *Global Burden of Disease and Injury Series* Vol. 1. Cambridge: Harvard School of Public Health on behalf of the World Health Organization and the World Bank, 1996.

Chapter 1 – Water

1. Ullah, H., et al. "Effects of Sugar, Salt and Distilled Water on White Blood Cells and Platelet Cells." *Journal of Tumor* 4 no. 1 (2015): 354-358.
2. Azoulay, A., Garzon, P., Eisenberg, M.J. "Comparison of the Mineral Content of Tap Water and Bottled Waters." *Journal of General Internal Medicine* 16 no. 3 (2001): 168-175.
3. Chuan, M.C., Shu, G.Y. "Solubility of Heavy Metals in a Contaminated Soil: Effects of Redox Potential and pH." *Water, Air, and Soil Pollution* 90 nos. 3-4 (1996): 543-556.
4. Kim, E.J., et al. "Effect of pH on the Concentrations of Lead and Trace Contaminants in Drinking Water; A Combined Batch, Pipe Loop and Sentinel Home Study." *Water Research* 45 no. 9 (2011): 2763-2774.
5. Payne, M. "Lead in Drinking Water." *Canadian Medical Association Journal* 179 no. 3 (2008): 253-254.
6. Sadiq, R., Rodriguez, M.J. "Disinfection By-products (DBPs) in Drinking Water and Predictive Models for their Occurrence: A Review." *Science of the Total Environment* 321 nos. 1-3 (2004): 21-46.
7. Schwalfenberg, G.K. "The Alkaline Diet: Is there Evidence that an Alkaline pH Diet Benefits Health?" *Journal of Environmental Public Health* (2012). Accessed June 29, 2017. doi: 727630.PMC.
8. Raveendran, R., Ashworth, B., Chatelier, B. "Manganese Removal in Drinking Water Systems." Presentation at the 64th annual water industry engineers and operators conference, September, 2001. 92-100.

9.   Deborde, M., Von Gunten, U.R.S. "Reactions of Chlorine with
      Inorganic and Organic Compounds during Water Treatment-Kinetics
      and Mechanisms: A Critical Review." *Water Research* 42, nos. 1-2
      (2008): 13-51.
10.   Dunnick, J.K., Melnick, R.L. "Assessment of the Carcinogenic
      Potential of Chlorinated Water: Experimental Studies of Chlorine,
      Chloramine, and Trihalomethanes." *Journal of the National Cancer
      Institute* 85, no. 10 (1993): 817-822. doi: 10.1093/jnci/85.10.817.
11.   S.D. Richardson, et. al., "Occurrence, Genotoxicity, and
      Carcinogenicity of Regulated and Emerging Disinfection By-
      products in Drinking Water: A Review and Roadmap for Research."
      Mutation Research/Reviews in Mutation Research 636 nos. 1-3
      (2007): 178-242. doi: 10.1016/j.mrrev.2007.09.001.
12.   Villanueva, C.M., et al. "Disinfection Byproducts and Bladder
      Cancer: A Pooled Analysis." *Epidemiology* 15 no. 3 (2004): 357-367.
      1. doi: 10.1097/01.ede.0000121380.02594.fc.
13.   World Health Organization. *Guidelines for drinking-water quality.*
      Vol. 1. Geneva: World Health Organization, 2004.
14.   Hood, E. "Tap Water and Trihalomethanes: Flow of Concerns
      Continues." *Environmental Health Perspectives* 133 no. 7 (2005):
      A474.
15.   Nuckols, J.R., et al. "Influence of Tap Water Quality and Household
      Water Use Activities on Indoor Air and Internal Dose Levels of
      Trihalomethanes." *Environmental Health Perspectives* 113 no. 7
      (2005): 863-870.
      2. doi: 10.1289/ehp.7141
16.   Jaishankar, M., et al. "Toxicity, Mechanism and Health Effects of
      Some Heavy Metals." *Interdisciplinary Toxicology* 7 no. 2 (2014):
      60-72.
      3. doi: 10.2478/intox-2014-0009.
17.   Sunitha, V., Reddy, B.M., Reddy, M.R. "Assessment of Groundwater
      Quality with Special Reference to Fluoride in South Eastern Part of
      Anantapur District, Andhra Pradesh." *Advances in Applied Science
      Research* 3 no. 3 (2012): 1618-1623.
18.   Yang, C.Y., et al. "Fluoride in Drinking Water and Cancer Mortality in
      Taiwan." *Environmental Research* 82 no. 3 (2000): 189-193. doi:
      10.1006/enrs.1999.4018.
19.   Cantor, K.P. "Drinking Water and Cancer." *Cancer Causes &
      Control* 8 no. 3 (1997): 292-308.
20.   Woolschlager J.E. "Water Quality Decay in Distribution Systems -
      Problems, Causes, and New Modeling Tools." *Urban Water Journal*
      2 no. 2 (2005): 69-79.
      4. doi: 10.1080/15730620500144027.
21.   Li, H., et al. "Effect of pH, Temperature, Dissolved Oxygen, and
      Flow Rate of Overlying Water on Heavy Metals Release from Storm
      Sewer Sediments." *Journal of Chemistry* 2013 (2013): Article ID
      434012, 11 pages.
      5. doi: 10.1155/2013/434012.
22.   Leijs, M.M., et al. "Thyroid Hormone Metabolism and Environmental
      Chemical Exposure." *Environmental Health* 11 no. 1 (2012): S10.
      6. doi: 10.1186/1476-069X-11-S1-S10.

23. Hsu, P.C., et al. "Airborne Persistent Organic Pollutants and Male Reproductive Health." *Aerosol and Air Quality Research* 14 (2014). 1292-1298.
7. doi: 10.4209/aaqr.2013.03.0066.
24. Srivastava, S., et al. "Testicular Toxicity of Di-N-Butyl Phthalate in Adult Rats: Effect on Marker Enzymes of Spermatogenesis." *Indian Journal of Experimental Biology* 28 no. 1 (1990). 67-70.
25. Steinmetz, R., et al. "The Environmental Estrogen Bisphenol A Stimulates Prolactin Release in Vitro and in Vivo. *Endocrinology* 138 no. 5 (1997). 1780-1786.
8. doi: 10.1210/endo.138.5.5132.
26. Steinmetz, R. et al. "The Xenoestrogen Bisphenol A Induces Growth, Differentiation, and c-fos Gene Expression in the Female Reproductive Tract." *Endocrinology* 139 no. 6 (1998). 2741-2747. doi: 10.1210/endo.139.6.6027.
27. Welshons, W.V., Nagel, S.C., vom Saal, F.S. "Large Effects from Small Exposures. III. Endocrine Mechanisms Mediating Effects of Bisphenol A at Levels of Human Exposure." *Endocrinology* 147 no. 7 (2006). s56-s69. doi: 10.1210/en.2005-1159.
28. Rochester, J.R., Bolden, A.L. "Bisphenol S and F: A Systematic Review and Comparison of the Hormonal Activity of Bisphenol A Substitutes." *Environmental Health Perspectives* 123 no. 7 (2015). doi: 10.1289/ehp.1408989.
29. Biles J.E., et. al. "Determination of bisphenol-A in Reusable Polycarbonate Food-contact Plastics and Migration to Food Simulating Liquids. *Journal of Agriculture and Food Chemistry* 45 (1997). 3541–3544. doi: 1021/jf970072i.
30. Al-Degs, Y.S., et al. "Effect of Solution pH, Ionic Strength, and Temperature on Adsorption Behavior of Reactive Dyes on Activated Carbon." *Dyes and Pigments* 77 no. 1 (2008). 16-23. doi: 10.1016/j.dyepig.2007.03.001.
31. Adams, M. "Water Filters Tested for Heavy Metals Removal: Zero Water, Pur, Brita, Mavea, Culligan, Seychelle and Waterman." *NaturalNews.com.* Accessed July 2, 2017. http://www.naturalnews.com/046536_water_filters_heavy_metals_lab_results.html
32. Michen B., et al. "Virus Removal in Ceramic Depth Filters Based on Diatomaceous Earth." *Environmental Science & Technology* 46 no. 2 (2012). 1170-1177.
9. doi: 10.1021/es2030565.
33. Li, D., Wang, H. "Recent Developments in Reverse Osmosis Desalination Membranes." *Journal of Materials Chemistry* 22 (2010). 4551-4566.
10. doi: 10.1039/B924553G.
34. Payment, P. et al. "Gastrointestinal Health Effects Associated with the Consumption of Drinking Water Produced by Point-of-use Domestic Reverse-osmosis Filtration Units." *Applied and Environmental Microbiology* 57 no. 4 (1991): 945-948. PMCID: PMC 182827.
35. Morita S., et al. "Efficacy of UV Irradiation in Inactivating *Cryptosporidium parvum* Oocysts." *Applied and Environmental*

Microbiology 68 no. 11 (2002). 5387-5393. doi:
10.1128/AEM.68.11.5387-5393.2002.

36.   Urbano dos Santos, L., et al. "Infectivity of *Giardia duodenalis* Cysts
      from UV Light-Disinfected Wastewater Effluent Using a Nude
      BALB/c Mouse Model." *ISRN Parasitology*, Jan 14, 2013. Accessed
      July 2, 2017.
      11. doi: 10.5402/2013/713958.

37.   Kozisek, F. "Health Risks from Drinking Demineralised Water:
      Nutrients in Drinking Water." Geneva: World Health Organization,
      2005.

38.   Yamabhai, M., et al. "Diverse Biological Effects of Electromagnetic-
      treated Water." *Homeopathy* 103 no. 3 (2014). 186-192. doi:
      10.1016/j.homp.2013.11.004.

Chapter 2 – Air

1.   Stucker, M., et al. "The Cutaneous Uptake of Atmospheric Oxygen
      Contributes Significantly to the Oxygen Supply of Human Dermis
      and Epidermis." *The Journal of Physiology* 538 pt. 3 (2002). 985-
      994. doi: 10.1113/jphysiol.2001.013067.

2.   Fellin, P., Otson, R. "Assessment of the Influence of Climatic
      Factors on Concentration Levels of Volatile Organic Compounds
      (VOCs) in Canadian Homes." *Atmospheric Environment* 28 no. 22
      (1994). 3581-3586.
      12. doi: 10.1016/1352-2310(94)00204-X.

3.   Bernstein, J.A., et al. "The Health Effects of Nonindustrial Indoor Air
      Pollution." *Journal of Allergy and Clinical Immunology* 121 no. 3
      (2008). 585-591.
      13. doi: 10.1016/j.jaci.2007.10.045.

4.   Zhang, J., Smith, K.R. "Indoor Air Pollution: A Global Health
      Concern." *British Medical Bulletin* 68 no.1 (2003). 209-225. doi:
      10.1093/bmb/ldg029.

5.   Pope, C.A., et al. "Lung Cancer, Cardiopulmonary Mortality, and
      Long Term Exposure to Fine Particulate Air Pollution." *Journal of the
      American Medical Association* 287 no. 9 (2002). 1132-1141.
      PMCID: PMC4037163.

6.   Robertson, A., et al. "The Cellular and Molecular Carcinogenic
      Effects of Radon Exposure: A Review." *International Journal of
      Molecular Sciences* 14 no.7 (2013): 14024-14063. doi:
      10.3390/ijms140714024.

7.   Quinn, D.K., et al. "Complications of Carbon Monoxide Poisoning: A
      Case Discussion and Review of the Literature." *The Primary Care
      Companion to the Journal of Clinical Psychiatry* 11 no. 2 (2009): 74-
      79. PMCID: PMC2707118.

8.   Girman, J.R., et al. "Causes of Unintentional Deaths from Carbon
      Monoxide Poisonings in California." *Western Journal of Medicine*
      168 (1998): 158-165.

9.   Lau, et al. "Levels of Selected Organic Compounds in Materials for
      Candle Production and Human Exposure to Candle Emissions."
      Chemosphere 34 nos. 5-7 (1997): 1623-1630.

10. Feng, Z., et al. "Acrolein is a Major Cigarette-related Lung Cancer Agent: Preferential Binding at *p53* Mutational Hotspots and Inhibition of DNA Repair." *Proceedings of the National Academy of Sciences of the United State of America* 103 no. 42 (2006): 15404-15409. doi: 10.1073/pnas.0607031103.

11. Isaxon, et al. "Contribution of Indoor-generated Particles to Residential Exposure." *Atmospheric Environment* 106 (2015): 458-466.
14. doi: 10.1016/ j.atmosenv.2014.07.053.

12. Nriagu J.O., Kim, M.J. "Emissions of Lead and Zinc from Candles with Metal-core Wicks." *Science of the Total Environment* 250 (2000): 31-37.

13. Lofroth, G., Stensman, C., and Brandhorst-Satzkorn, M. "Indoor Sources of Mutagenic Aerosol Particulate Matter: Smoking, Cooking, and Incense Burning." *Mutation Research* 261 (1991): 21-28.

14. Orechio, S., et al. "Volatile Profiles of Emissions from Different Activities Analyzed Using Canister Samplers and GAs Chromatography-Mass Spectrometry (GC/MS) Analysis: A Case Study." *International Journal Environmental Research and Public Health* 14 no. 2 (2017): 195. Accessed July 6, 2017.
15. doi: 10.3390/ijerph14020195.

15. Derudi, M., et al. "Emission of Air Pollutants from Burning Candles with Different Composition in Indoor Environments." *Environmental Science Pollution Research International* 21 no. 6 (2014): 4320-4330. doi: 10.1007/s11356-013-2394-2.

16. Naeem, Z. "Second-hand Smoke - Ignored Implications." *International Journal of Health Sciences (Qassim)* 9 no. 2 (2015): V-VI. PMCID: PMC4538886.

17. Callahan-Lyon, P. "Electronic Cigarettes: Human Health Effects." *Tobacco Control* 23 (2014): ii36-ii40.

18. Leigh, N.J., et al. "Flavourings Significantly Affect Inhalation Toxicity of Aerosol Generated from Electronic Nicotine Delivery Systems (ENDS)." *Tobacco Control* 25 (2016): ii81-ii87.

19. Flora, G., Gupta, D., and Tiwari, A. "Toxicity of Lead: A Review with Recent Updates." *Interdisciplinary Toxicology* 5 no. 2 (2012): 47-58.
16. doi: 10.2478/v10102-012-0009-2.

20. Hou, S., et al. "A Clinical Study of the Effects of Lead Poisoning on the Intelligence and Neurobehavioral Abilities of Children." *Theoretical Biology and Medical Modelling* 10 no. 13 (2013). Accessed July 6, 2017.
17. doi: 10.1186/1742-4682-10-13.

21. Flannagan, P.R., Chamberlain, M.J., Valberg, L.S. "The Relationship Between Iron and Lead Absorption in Humans." *American Journal of Clinical Nutrition* 36 no. 5 (1982): 823-829.

22. Blake, K.C.H., Mann, M. "Effect of Calcium and Phosphorus on the Gastrointestinal Absorption of 203Pb in Man." *Environmental Research* 30 no. 1 (1983): 188-194.

23. Salthammer, T., Mentese, S., Marutzky, R. "Formaldehyde in the Indoor Environment." *Chemical Reviews* 110 no. 4 (2010): 2536-2572.

18. doi: 10.1021/cr800399g.

24. Hauptmann, M., et al. "Mortality from Solid Cancers Among Workers in Formaldehyde Industries." *American Journal of Epidemiology* 159 no. 12 (2004): 1117-1130.

25. Dingle, P., Tan, R., Cheong, C. "Formaldehyde in Occupied and Unoccupied Caravans in Australia." *Indoor Built Environment* 9 (2000): 233-236.
     19. doi: 10.1159/000057512.

26. Snyder, F., "Leukemia and Benzene." *International Journal of Environmental Research and Public Health* 9 no. 8 (2012): 2875-2893.
     20. doi: 10.3390/ijerph9082875.

27. Rice, J.M., et al. "Rodent Tumors of Urinary Bladder, Renal Cortex, and Thyroid Gland in IARC Monographs Evaluations of Carcinogenic Risk to Humans." *Toxicological Sciences* 49 (1999): 166-171.

28. Hession, R.M., et al. "Multiple Sclerosis Disease Progression and Paradichlorobenzene - A Tale of Mothballs and Toilet Cleaner." *Journal of the American Medical Association Neurology* 71 no. 2 (2014): 228-232.
     21. doi: 10.1001/jamaneurol.2013.4395.

29. Schumann, A.M., Quast, J.F., Watanabe, P.G. "The Pharmacokinetics and Macromolecular Interactions of Perchloroethylene in Mice and Rats as Related to Oncogenicity." *Toxicology and Applied Pharmacology* 55 no. 2 (1980): 207-219.

30. Raaschou-Nielsen, O., et al. "Cancer Risk Among Workers at Danish Companies Using Trichloroethylene: A Cohort Study." *Society for Epidemiologic Research* 158 no. 12 (2003): 1182-1192. doi: 10.1093/aje/kwg282.

31. Zain, M.E. "Impact of Mycotoxins on Humans and Animals." *Journal of Saudi Chemical Society* 15 no. 2 (2011): 129-144. doi: 10.1016/j.jscs.2010.06.006.

32. Hope, J., "A Review of the Mechanism of Injury and Treatment Approaches for Illness Resulting from Exposure to Water-Damaged Buildings, Mold, and Mycotoxins." *The Scientific World Journal* 2013 (2013): 20 pages. doi: 10.1155/2013/767482.

33. Kuhn, D.M., Ghannoum, M.A. "Indoor Mold, Toxigenic Fungi, and *Stachybotrys chartarum*: Infectious Disease Perspective." *Clinical Microbiology Reviews* 16 no. 1 (2003): 144-172. doi: 10.1128/CMR.16.1.144-172.2003.

34. Lantz, P.M., Mendez, D., Philbert, M.A. "Radon, Smoking, and Lung Cancer: The Need to Refocus Radon Control Policy." *American Journal of Public Health* 103 no. 3 (2013): 443-447. doi: 10.2105/AJPH.2012.300926.

35. "A Citizen's Guide to Radon: The Guide to Protecting Yourself and Your Family from Radon." EPA 402/K-09/011. *EPA.gov.* January 2009. Accessed July 8, 2017. https://www.epa.gov/sites/production/files/2016-02/documents/2012_a_citizens_guide_to_radon.pdf.

36. Jensen, H.K., et al. "Pesticide Use and Self-Reported Symptoms of Acute Pesticide Poisoning Among Aquatic Farmers in Phnom Penh,

Cambodia." *Journal of Toxicology* Volume 2011 (2011): Accessed July 8, 2017. 8 pages. doi: 10.1155/2011/639814.

37. Hu, R., et al. "Long- and Short-Term Health Effects of Pesticide Exposure: A Cohort Study from China." *PLOS ONE.* June 4, 2015. Accessed July 8, 2017. doi: 10.1371/journal.pone.0128766.

38. Bassil, K.L., et al. "Cancer Health Effects of Pesticides: Systematic Review." *Canadian Family Physician* 53 no. 10 (2007): 1704-1711. PMCID: PMC2231435.

39. Brunekreef, B., Forsberg, B. "Epidemiological Evidence of Effects of Coarse Airborne Particles on Health." *European Respiratory Journal* 26 (2005): 309-318. doi: 10.1183/09031936.05.00001805.

40. Brook, R.D., et al. "Particulate Matter Air Pollution and Cardiovascular Disease: An Update to the Scientific Statement from the American Heart Association." *Circulation* 121 no. 21 (2010): 2331-2378. doi: 10.1161/CIR.0b013e3181dbece1.

41. Zhao, D., Azimi, P., Stephens, B. "Evaluating the Long-Term Health and Economic Impacts of Central Residential Air Filtration for Reducing Premature Mortality Associated with Indoor Fine Particulate Matter ($PM_{2.5}$) of Outdoor Origin." *International Journal of Environmental Research and Public Health* 12 no. 7 (2015): 8448-8479. doi: 10.3390/ijerph120708448.

42. Sublett, J.L. "Effectiveness of Air Filters and Air Cleaners in Allergic Respiratory Diseases: A Review of the Recent Literature." *Current Allergy and Asthma Reports* 11 no. 5 (2011): 395-402. doi: 10.1007/s11882-011-0208-5.

43. Joshi, S.M. "The Sick Building Syndrome." *Indian Journal of Occupational & Environmental Medicine* 12 no. 2 (2008): 61-64. doi: 10.4103/0019-5278.43262.

44. Mosaddegh, M.H., et al. "Phytoremediation of Benzene, Toluene, Ethylbenzene and Xylene Contaminated Air by *D. deremensis* and *O. microdasys* plants." *Journal of Environmental Health Science and Engineering* 12 no. 39 (2014). Accessed July 8, 2017. doi: 10.1186/2052-336X-12-39.

45. Wolverton, B.C., Wolverton, J.D. "Plants and Soil Microorganisms: Removal of Formaldehyde, Xylene, and Ammonia from the Indoor Environment." *Journal of the Mississippi Academy of Sciences* 38 no. 2 (1993): 11-15.

46. Yang, D.S., et al. "Screening Indoor Plants for Volatile Organic Pollutant Removal Efficiency." *Horticulture Science* 44 no. 5 (2009): 1377-1381.

47. Krueger, A.P., Reed, E.J. "Biological Impact of Small Air Ions." *Science* 193 (1976): 1209-1213. PMID: 959834.

48. Dowdall, M., De Montigny, C. "Effect of Atmospheric Ions on Hippocampal Pyramidal Neuron Responsiveness to Serotonin." *Brain Research* 342 (1985): 103-109.

49. Pino, O., La Ragione, F. "There's Something in the Air: Empirical Evidence for the Effects of Air Ions (NAI) on Psychophysiological State and Performance." *Research in Psychology and Behavioral Sciences* 1 no. 4 (2013): 48-53. doi: 10.12691/rpbs-1-4-1.

50.   Hawkins, L.H., Barker, T. "Air Ions and Human Performance."
       Ergonomics 21 no. 4 (1978): 273-278. doi:
       10.1080/00140137808931724.
51.   Wallner, P., et al. "Exposure to Air Ions in Indoor Environments:
       Experimental Study with Healthy Adults." *International Journal of
       Environmental Research and Public Health* 12 no. 11 (2015):
       14301-14311. doi: 10.3390/ijerph121114301.
52.   Harmer, C.J., et al. "Negative Ion Treatment Increases Positive
       Emotional Processing in Seasonal Affective Disorder."
       Psychological Medicine 42 no. 8 (2012): 1605-1612. doi:
       10.1017/S0033291711002820.
53.   Terman, M., Terman, J.S., Ross, D.C. "A Controlled Trial of Timed
       Bright Light and Negative Air Ionization for Treatment of Winter
       Depression." *Archives of General Psychiatry* 55 no. 10 (1998): 875-
       882. doi: 10.1001/archpsyc.55.10.875.
54.   Gallo, C.F., Lama, W.L. "Some Charge Exchange Phenomena
       Explained by a Classical Model of the Work Function." *Journal of
       Electrostatics* 2 no. 2 (1976): 145-150. doi: 10.1016/0304-
       3886(76)90005-X.
55.   Ling, X., Jayaratne, R., Morawska, L. "Air Ion Concentrations in
       Various Urban Outdoor Environments." *Atmospheric Environment*
       44 no. 18 (2010): 2186-2193. doi: 10.1016/j.atmosenv.2010.03.026.
56.   Hawkins, L.H. "The Influence of Air Ions, Temperature and Humidity
       on Subjective Wellbeing and Comfort." *Journal of Environmental
       Psychology* 1 no. 4 (1981): 279-292. doi:10.1016/S0272-
       4944(81)80026-6.
57.   Ali, B., et al. "Essential Oils Used in Aromatherapy: A Systemic
       Review." *Asian Pacific Journal of Tropical Biomedicine* 5 no. 8
       (2015): 601-611. doi: 10.1016/j.apjtb.2015.05.007.
58.   Silva-Neto, R.P., Peres, M.F., Valenca, M.M. "Odorant Substances
       that Trigger Headaches in Migraine Patients." *Cephalalgia* 34
       (2014): 14-21.
59.   Potera, C. "INDOOR AIR QUALITY: Scented Products Emit a
       Bouquet of VOCs." *Environmental Health Perspectives* 119 no. 1
       (2011): A16. Accessed July 8, 2017. doi: 10.1289/ehp.119-a16.

Chapter 3 – Whole Food

1.   Marchesi, J.R. et al. "The Gut Microbiota and Host Health: a New
       Clinical Frontier." *Gut.* September 2, 2015. Accessed July 9, 2017.
       doi: 10.1136/gutjnl-2015-309990.
2.   Amvrazi, E.G. "Fate of Pesticide Residues on Raw Agricultural
       Crops After Postharvest Storage and Food Processing to Edible
       Portions." In *Pesticides – Formulations, Effects, Fate,* ed. Margarita
       Stoytcheva. *InTech* (2011): Chapter 28.
       29. doi: 10.5772/13988.
3.   Angioni, A. et al. "Residues of Azoxystrobin, Fenhexamid and
       Pyrimethanil in Strawberry Following Field Treatments and the
       Effect of Domestic Washing." *Food Additives and Contaminants* 21
       (2004): 1065-1070.

4.   Kong, Z, et al. "Effect of Home Processing on the Distribution and
      Reduction of Pesticide Residues in Apples." *Food Additives &*
      Contaminants: Part A 29 no. 8 (2012): 1280-1287. doi:
      10.1080/19440049.2012.690347.
5.   Reynolds, P., et al. "Childhood Cancer and Agricultural Pesticide
      Use, an Ecologic Study in California." *Environmental Health*
      Perspectives 110 no. 3 (2002): 319-324.
6.   Mnif, W., et al. "Effect of Endocrine Disruptor Pesticides: A Review."
      International Journal of Environmental Research and Public Health
      8 no. 6 (2011): 2265-2303. doi: 10.3390/ijerph8062265.
7.   London, L., et al. "Neurobehavioral and Neurodevelopmental Effects
      of Pesticide Exposures." *Neurotoxicology* 33 no. 4 (2012): 887-896.
      30. doi 10.1016/j.neuro.2012.01.004.
8.   Council on Environmental Health. "Pesticide Exposure in Children."
      Pediatrics December 2012.
9.   Sears, M.E., Genuis, S.J. "Environmental Determinants of Chronic
      Disease and Medical Approaches: Recognition, Avoidance,
      Supportive Therapy, and Detoxification." *Journal of Environmental*
      and Public Health 2012 (2012): Article ID 356798, 15 pages. doi:
      10.1155/2012/356798.
10.   Snedeker, S.M., Hay, A.G. "Do Interactions Between Gut Ecology
      and Environmental Chemicals Contribute to Obesity and Diabetes?"
      Environmental Health Perspectives 120 no. 3 (2012): 332-339.
11.   "Adoption of Genetically Engineered Crops in the U.S." *United*
      States Department of Agriculture Economic Research Service. Last
      modified July 14, 2016. Accessed July 9, 2017.
12.   Zobiole, L.H.S., Kremer, R.J., de Oliveira, R.S. "Glyphosate
      Interactions with Physiological, Microbiological, and Nutritional
      Parameters in Glyphosate-Resistant Soybeans." In *Soybeans:*
      Cultivation, Uses and Nutrition, ed. Jason Maxwell (2011): 251-272.
13.   Johal, G.S., Huber, D.M. "Glyphosate Effects on Diseases of
      Plants." *European Journal of Agronomy* 31 no. 3 (2009): 144-152.
      doi: 10.1016/j.eja.2009.04.004.
14.   Arregui, M.C., et al. "Monitoring Glyphosate Residues in Transgenic
      Glyphosate-resistant Soybean." *Pest Management Science* 60
      (2004):163-166.
      31. doi: 10.1002/ps.775.
15.   Monsanto Technology LLC. "Glyphosate Formulations and their use
      for the Inhibition of 5-enolpyruvylshikimate-3-phosphate Synthase."
      Accessed July 9, 2017. Missouri: Monsanto Technology LLC, 2010.
      https://www.google.com/patents/US7771736.
16.   Camran, J.A., et al. "A Long-Term Toxicology Study on Pigs Fed a
      Combined Genetically Modified (GM) Soy and GM Maize Diet."
      Journal of Organic Systems 8 no. 1 (2013): 38-54.
17.   Shehata, A.A., et al. "The Effect of Glyphosate on Potential
      Pathogens and Beneficial Members of Poultry Microbiota in Vitro."
      Current Microbiology 66 no. 4 (2013): 350-358. doi:
      10.1007/s00284-012-0277-2.
18.   Round, J.L., Mazmanian, S.K. "The Gut Microbiome Shapes
      Intestinal Immune Responses During Health and Disease." *National*

Reviews Immunology 9 no. 5, (2009): 313-323. doi:
10.1038/nri2515.

19.   Samsel, A., Seneff S. "Glyphosate, Pathways to Modern Diseases
       II: Celiac Sprue and Gluten Intolerance." *Interdisciplinary
       Toxicology.* 6 no. 4 (2013): 159-184.
       32. doi: 10.2478/intox-2013-0026.

20.   Vasiluk, L., Pinto, L.J., Moore, M.M. "Oral Bioavailability of
       Glyphosate: Studies Using Two Intestinal Cell Lines." *Environmental
       Toxicology* (2005). Accessed July 9, 2017. doi: 10.1897/04-088R.1.

21.   Kruger, M., et al. "Detection of Glyphosate Residues in Animals and
       Humans." *Environmental & Analytical Toxicology* 4 no. 2 (2014).
       Accessed July 9, 2017.
       33. doi: 10.4172/2161-0525.1000210.

22.   Gasnier, C., et al. "Glyphosate-Based Herbicides are Toxic and
       Endocrine Disruptors in Human Cell Lines." *Toxicology* 262 no. 3
       (2009): 184-191.
       34. doi: 10.1016/j.tox.2009.06.006.

23.   Thongprakaisang, S., et al. "Glyphosate Induces Human Breast
       Cancer Cells Growth via Estrogen Receptors." *Food and Chemical
       Toxicology* 59 (2013): 129-136. doi: 10.1016/j.fct.2013.05.057.

24.   U.S. Government Accountability Office. "FOOD SAFETY: FDA and
       USDA Should Strengthen Pesticide Residue Monitoring Programs
       and Further Disclose Monitoring Limitations." (2014): 15-38.
       Accessed July 9, 2017. U.S. Government Accountability Office.

25.   Mostafalou, S., Abdollahi, M. "Pesticides and Human Chronic
       Diseases: Evidences, Mechanisms, and Perspectives." *Toxicology
       and Applied Pharmacology* 268 no. 2 (2013): 157-177. doi:
       10.1016/j.taap.2013.01.025.

26.   Ribas, G., et al. "Genotoxicity of the Herbicides Alachlor and Maleic
       Hydrazide in Cultured Human Lymphocytes." *Mutagenesis* 11 no. 3
       (1996): 221-227.
       35. doi: 10.1093/mutage/11.3.221.

27.   Lee, W.C., et al. "High Performance Liquid Chromatographic
       Determination of Maleic Hydrazide Residue in Potatoes." *Journal of
       Food and Drug Analysis* 9 no. 3 (2001): 167-172.

28.   Shibamoto, T., Bjeldanes, L.F. "Natural Toxins in Plant Foodstuffs."
       in *Introduction to Food Toxicology*. San Diego: Academic Press,
       1993. 78-79, 82-84.

29.   Potera, C. "DIET AND NUTRITION: The Artificial Food Dye Blues."
       Environmental Health Perspectives 118 no. 10 (2010): A428.
       Accessed July 9, 2017.
       36. doi: 10.1289/ehp.118-a428.

30.   Food Standards Agency. *Compulsory Warnings on Colours in Food
       and Drink.* [press release] London: Food Standards Agency, July 22,
       2010. Accessed July 9, 2017. http://tinyurl.com/2d44wlz.

31.   Bajwa, U., Sandhu, K.S. "Effect of Handling and Processing on
       Pesticide Residues in Food – a Review." *Journal of Food Science
       and Technology* 51 no. 2 (2014): 201-220. doi: 10.1007/s13197-
       011-0499-5.

32.   Lee, M.G., Lee, S.R. "Reduction Factors and Risk Assessment of Organophosphorus Pesticides in Korean Foods." *Korean Journal of Food Science Technology* 29 (1997): 240-248.

33.   Koseki, S., Itoh, K. "Effect of Nitrogen Gas Packaging on the Quality and Microbial Growth of Fresh-cut Vegetables Under Low Temperatures." *Journal of Food Protection* 65 no. 2 (2002): 326-332. PMID: 11848563.

34.   Monk, J.D., Beuchat, L.R., Doyle, M.P. "Irradiation Inactivation of Food-Borne Microorganisms." *Journal of Food Protection* 58 no. 2 (1995): 197-208.
      37. doi: 10.4315/0362-028X-58.2.197.

35.   Petursdottir, A.H., Sloth, J.J., Feldmann, J. "Introduction of Regulations for Arsenic in Feed and Food with Emphasis on Inorganic Arsenic, and Implications for Analytical Chemistry." *Analytical and Bioanalytical Chemistry* 407 no. 28, (2015): 8385-8396. doi: 10.1007/s00216-015-9019-1.

36.   Ferguson, D.M., Warner, R.D. "Have We Underestimated the Impact of Pre-slaughter Stress on Meat Quality in Ruminants?" *Meat Science* 80 no. 1 (2008): 12-19. doi: 10.1016/j.meatsci.2008.05.004.

37.   US Department of Health and Human Services, Public Health Service. *Toxicological Profile for Mercury*. Atlanta: US Department of Health and Human Services, 1999.

38.   Rice, K.M., et al. "Environmental Mercury and its Toxic Effects." *Journal of Preventive Medical Public Health* 47 no. 2 (2014): 74-83.
      38. doi: 0.3961/jpmph.2014.47.2.74.

39.   Myers, G.J., Davidson, P.W., Strain, J.J. "Nutrient and Methyl Mercury Exposure from Consuming Fish." *The Journal of Nutrition* 137 no. 12 (2007): 2805-2808.

40.   Environmental Protection Agency. "EPA-FDA Advice about Eating Fish and Shellfish." Environmental Protection Agency, 2017. Accessed July 10, 2017. https://www.epa.gov/fish-tech/2017-epa-fda-advice-about-eating-fish-and-shellfish.

41.   Hites, R.A., et al. "Global Assessment of Polybrominated Diphenyl Ethers in Farmed and Wild Salmon." *Environmental Science & Technology* 38 no. 19 (2004): 4945-4949. doi: 10.1021/es049548m.

42.   Pirkle, J.L., et al. "Estimates of the Half-Life of 2,3,7,8-tetrachlorodibenzo-p-dioxin in Vietnam Veterans of Operation Ranch Hand." *Journal of Toxicology and Environmental Health* 27 no. 2 (1989): 165-171.
      39. doi: 10.1080/15287398909531288.

43.   Fry, J.P., et al. "Environmental Health impacts of Feeding Crops to Farmed Fish." *Environment International* 91 (2016): 201-214. doi: 10.1016/j.envint.2016.02.022.

44.   Buschmann, A.H., et al. "Salmon Aquaculture and Antimicrobial Resistance in the Marine Environment." *PLOS ONE* (August 8, 2012).
      40. doi: 10.1371/journal.pone.0042724.

45.   Silbernagel, S.M., et al. "Recognizing and Preventing Overexposure to Methylmercury from Fish and Seafood Consumption: Information for Physicians." *Journal of Toxicology* 2011 (2011): 983072.
      41. doi: 10.1155/2011/983072.

46.   Filipkowska, A., Lubecki, L. "Endocrine Disruptors in Blue Mussels
      and Sediments from the Gulf of Gdansk (Southern Baltic)."
      Environmental Science Pollution Research 23 (2016): 13864-13876.
      doi: 10.1007/s11356-016-6524-5.
47.   Rodriguez-Hernandez, A., et al. "Comparative Study of the Intake of
      Toxic Persistent and Semi Persistent Pollutants Through the
      Consumption of Fish and Seafood from Two Modes of Production
      (Wild-caught and Farmed)." *Science of the Total Environment* 575
      no. 1 (2017): 919-931.
48.   Vass, M., Hruska, K., Franek, M. "Nitrofuran Antibiotics: a Review
      on the Application, Prohibition and Residual Analysis." *Veterinarni
      Medicina* 53 no. 9 (2008): 469-500.
49.   Hassan, M.N. et al. "Monitoring the Presence of Chloramphenicol
      and Nitrofuran Metabolites in Cultured Prawn, Shrimp and Feed in
      the Southwest Coastal Region of Bangladesh." *The Egyptian
      Journal of Aquatic Research* 39 no. 1 (2013): 51-58.
50.   MacDonald, L.E., et al. "A Systematic Review and Meta-Analysis of
      the Effects of Pasteurization on Milk Vitamins, and Evidence for
      Raw Milk Consumption and Other Health-Related Outcomes."
      Journal of Food Protection 74 no. 11 (2011): 1814-1832. doi:
      10.4315/0362-028X.JFP-10-269.
51.   Gould, L.H., Mungai, E., Behravesh, C.B. "Outbreaks Attributed to
      Cheese: Differences Between Outbreaks Caused by Unpasteurized
      and Pasteurized Dairy Products, United States, 1998-2011."
      Foodborne Pathogenic Disease 11 no. 7 (2014): 545-551. doi:
      10.1089/fpd.2013.1650.
52.   alKanhal, H.A., al-Othman, A.A., Hewedi, F.M. "Changes in Protein
      Nutritional Quality in Fresh and Recombined Ultra High
      Temperature Treated Milk During Storage." *International Journal of
      Food Science Nutrition* 52 no. 6 (2001): 509-514. PMID: 11570017.
53.   "Recombinant Bovine Growth Hormone." *American Cancer Society*,
      a, https://www.cancer.org/cancer/cancer-causes/recombinant-
      bovine-growth-hormone.html.
54.   Ganmaa, D., Sato A. "The Possible Role of Female Sex Hormones
      in Milk from Pregnant Cows in the Development of Breast, Ovarian
      and Corpus Uteri Cancers." *Medical Hypotheses* 65 no. 6 (2005):
      1028-1037.
      42. doi: 10.1016/j.mehy.2005.06.026.
55.   Lu, W., et al. "Dairy Products Intake and Cancer Mortality Risk: a
      Meta-Analysis of 11 Population-Based Cohort Studies." *Nutrition
      Journal* 15 no. 91 (2016). Accessed July 11, 2017. doi:
      10.1186/s12937-016-0210-9.
56.   Dohoo, I.R., et al. "A Meta-Analysis Review of the Effects of
      Recombinant Bovine Somatotropin: 2. Effects on Animal Health,
      Reproductive Performance, and Culling." *Canadian Journal of
      Veterinary Research.* 67 no. 4 (2003): 252-264.
57.   US Department of Agriculture. "Dairy 2007 Part III: Reference of
      Dairy Cattle Health and Management Practices in the United States,
      2007." Fort Collins: USDA, 2007. Accessed July 7, 2011.
      http://www.aphis.usda.gov/animal_health/nahms/dairy/downloads/d
      airy07/Dairy07_dr_PartIII_rev.pdf.

58. Food and Drug Administration. "Milk Drug Residue Sampling Survey." March 2015. Accessed July 11, 2017. https://www.fda.gov/downloads/AnimalVeterinary/GuidanceComplia nceEnforcement/ComplianceEnforcement/UCM435759.pdf.

59. Landers, T.F., et al. "A Review of Antibiotic Use in Food Animals: Perspective, Policy, and Potential." *Public Health Reports* 127 no. 1 (2012): 4-22.
43. doi: 10.1177/003335491212700103.

60. Kruger, M., et al. "Glyphosate Suppresses the Antagonistic Effect of *Enterococcus spp.* on *Clostridium botulinum.*" *Anaerobe* 20 (2013): 74-78.

61. Shehata, A.A., et al. "The Effect of Glyphosate on Potential Pathogens and Beneficial Members of Poultry Microbiota In Vitro." *Current Microbiology* 66 no. 4 (2013): 350-358. doi: 10.1007/s00284-012-0277-2.

62. Bailey, J.S., Cosby, D.E. "Salmonella Prevalence in Free-Range and Certified Organic Chickens." *Journal of Food Protection* 68 no. 11 (2005): 2451-2453.
44. doi: 10.4315/0362-028X-68.11.2451.

63. Lam, S.K., Ng, T.B. "Lectins: Production and Practical Applications." *Applied Microbiology and Biotechnology* 89 no. 1 (2011): 45-55.
45. doi: 10.1007/s00253-010-2892-9.

64. Freed, D.L.J. "Do Dietary Lectins Cause Disease?" *British Medical Journal* 318 no. 7190 (1999): 1023-1024. PMID: PMC1115436.

65. Ballhorn, D.J., et al. "Cyanogenesis of Wild Lima Bean (*Phaseolus lunatus L.)* is an Efficient Direct Defence in Nature," *PLOS ONE* (May 8, 2009). Accessed July 11, 2017. doi: 10.1371/journal.pone.0005450.

66. Latifkar, M., Mojaddam, M., Nejad, T.S. "The Effect of Application Time of *Cycocel* Hormone and Plant Density on Yield and Yield Components of Wheat (Chamran cultivar) in Ahvaz Weather Conditions." *International Journal of Biosciences* 4 no. 10 (2014): 234-242.

67. Bresnahan, G.A., et al. "Glyphosate Applied Preharvest Induces Shikimic Acid Accumulation in Hard Red Spring Wheat (*Triicum aestivum*)." *Journal of Agriculture and Food Chemistry* 51 no. 14 (2003): 4004-4007.
46. doi: 10.1021/jf0301753.

68. Hernandez, A.F., et al. "Toxic Effects of Pesticide Mixtures at a Molecular Level: Their Relevance to Human Health." *Toxicology* 307 no. 10 (2013): 136-145.
47. doi: 10.1016/j.tox.2012.06.009.

69. Ripsin, C.M., et al. "Oat Products and Lipid Lowering: A Meta-analysis." *Journal of the American Medical Association* 267 no. 24 (1992): 3317-3325.
48. doi: 10.1001/jama.1992.03480240079039.

70. Nguyen, K.T.N., Ryu, D. "Concentration of Ochratoxin A in Breakfast Cereals and Snacks Consumed in the United States." *Food Control* 40 (2014): 140-144.
49. doi: 10.1001/jama.1992.03480240079039.

71.   Lee, H.J., Ruy, D. "Significance of Ochratoxin A in Breakfast Cereals from the United States." *Journal of Agriculture and Food Chemistry* 63 no. 43 (2015): 9404-9409. doi: 10.1021/jf505674v.
72.   Huang, Z., et al. "Health Risk Assessment of Heavy Metals in Rice to the Population in Zhejiang, China." *PLOS ONE* (September 6, 2013). Accessed July 11, 2017. doi: 10.1371/journal.pone.0075007.

Chapter 4 – Processed Food

1.   Cunha S.C., et al. "Determination of Bisphenol A and Bisphenol B in Canned Seafood Combining QuEcHERS Extraction with Dispersive Liquid-Liquid Microextraction Followed by Gas Chromatography-Mass Spectrometry." *Analytical and Bioanalytical Chemistry* 404 no. 8 (2012): 2453-2463. doi: 10.1007/s00216-012-6389-5.
2.   Munguia-Lopez, E.M., Soto-Valdez, H. "Effect of Heat Processing and Storage Time on Migration of Bisphenol A (BPA) and Bisphenol A-Diglycidyl Ether (BADGE) to Aqueous Food Simulant from Mexican Can Coatings." *Journal of Agriculture and Food Chemistry* 49 no. 8 (2001): 3666-3671. doi: 10.1021/jf0009044.
3.   Yang, C.Z., et al. "Most Plastic Products Release Estrogenic Chemicals: A Potential Health Problem that Can be Solved." *Environmental Health Perspectives* 119 no. 7 (2011): 989-996. doi: 10.1289/ehp.1003220.
4.   Viuda-Martos, M., et al. "Functional Properties of Honey, Propolis, and Royal Jelly." *Journal of Food Science* 73 (2008): R117-R124. Accessed July 11, 2017.
       50. doi: 10.1111/j.1750-3841.2008.00966.x.
5.   Geuns, J.M.C. "Stevioside." *Phytochemistry* 64 no. 5 (2003): 913-921.
       51. doi: 10.1016/S0031-9422(03)00426-6.
6.   Brahmachari, G., et al. "Stevioside and Related Compounds – Molecules of Pharmaceutical Promise: A Critical Overview." *Arch Pharm Chemistry in the Life Sciences* 1 (2011): 5-19. doi: 10.1002/ardp.201000181.
7.   Mortensen, A. "Sweeteners Permitted in the European Union: Safety Aspects." *Scandinavian Journal of Food and Nutrition* 50 no. 3 (2006): 104-116.
       52. doi: 10.1080/17482970600982719.
8.   Smeets, P.A.M., et al. "Functional Magnetic Resonance Imaging of Human Hypothalamic Responses to Sweet Taste and Calories." *American Journal of Clincial Nutrition* 82 (2005): 1011-1016.
9.   Fowler, S.P. "Fueling the Obesity Epidemic? Artificially Sweetened Beverage Use and Long-term Weight Gain." *Obesity* 16 (2008): 1894-1900.
       53. doi: 10.1038/oby.2008.284.
10.   Soffritti, M., et al. "First Experimental Demonstration of the Multipotential Carcinogenic Effects of Aspartame Administered in the Feed to Sprague-Dawley Rats." *Environmental Health Perspectives* 114 no. 3 (2006): 379-385.
       54. PMCID: PMC1392232.

11. Tandel, K.R. "Sugar Substitutes: Health Controversy over Perceived Benefits." *Journal of Pharmacology & Pharmacotherapeutics* 2 no. 4 (2011): 236-243.
    55. doi: 10.4103/0976-500X.85936.
12. Parker, K., Salas, M., Nwosu, V.C. "High Fructose Corn Syrup: Production, Uses and Public Health Concerns." *Biotechnology and Molecular Biology Review* 5 no. 5 (2010): 71-78.
13. Schaefer, E.J., Gleason, J.A., Dansinger, M.L. "Dietary Fructose and Glucose Differentially Affect Lipid and Glucose Homeostasis." *The Journal of Nutrition* 13 no. 6 (2009): 1257S-1262S. doi: 10.3945/jn.108.098186.
14. Charrez, B., Qiao, L., Hebbard, L. "The Role of Fructose in Metabolism and Cancer." *Hormone Molecular Biology and Clinical Investigation* 22 no. 2 (2015): 79-89. doi: 10.1515/hmbci-2015-0009.
15. Rapin, J.R., Wiernsperger, N. "Possible Links between Intestinal Permeability and Food Processing: A Potential Therapeutic Niche for Glutamine." *Clinics* 65 no. 6 (2010): 635-643. doi: 10.1590/S1807-59322010000600012.
16. O'Keefe, J.H., Cordain, L. "Cardiovascular Disease Resulting From a Diet and Lifestyle at Odds with our Paleolithic Genome: How to Become a 21st Century Hunter-Gatherer." *Mayo Clinic Proceedings* 79 no. 1 (2004): 101-108.
    56. doi: 10.4065/79.1.101.
17. Dufault, R., et al. "Mercury from Chlor-Alkali Plants: Measured Concentrations in Product Sugar." *Environmental Health* 8 no. 2 (2009). Accessed July 12, 2017.
    57. doi: 10.1186/1476-069X-8-2.
18. Freston, J.W., et al. "Review and Analysis of the Effects of Olestra, a Dietary Fat Substitute, on Gastrointestinal Function and Symptoms." *Regulatory Toxicology and Pharmacology* 26 no. 2 (1997): 210-218. doi: 10.1006/rtph.1997.1165.
19. Schlagheck, T.G., et al. "Olestra Dose Response on Fat-Soluble and Water-Soluble Nutrients in Humans." *The Journal of Nutrition* 127 no. 8 (1997): 1646S-1665S. Accessed July 13, 2017.
20. Lopez-Garcia, E., et al. "Consumption of Trans Fatty Acids is Related to Plasma Biomarkers of Inflammation and Endothelial Dysfunction." *The Journal of Nutrition* 135 no. 3 (2005): 562-566.
21. Dhaka, V., et al. "Trans Fats – Sources, Health Risks and Alternative Approach – A Review." *Journal of Food Science Technology* 48 no. 5 (2011): 534-541.
    58. doi: 10.1007/s13197-010-0225-8.
22. Hunter, J.E., Zhang, J., Kris-Etherton, P.M. "Cardiovascular Disease Risk of Dietary Stearic Acid Compared with Trans, Other Saturated, and Unsaturated Fatty Acids: a Systematic Review." *The American Journal of Clinical Nutrition* 91 no. 1 (2010): 46-63. doi: 10.3945/ajcn.2009.27661.
23. Milkowski, A., et al. "Nutritional Epidemiology in the Context of Nitric Oxide Biology: A Risk-Benefit Evaluation for Dietary Nitrite and Nitrate." *Nitric Oxide* 22 no. 3 (2010): 110-119. doi: 10.1016/j.niox.2009.08.004.

24.   Bingham, S.A., et al. "Does Increased Endogenous Formation of *N*-Nitroso Compounds in the Human Colon Explain the Association Between Red Meat and Colon Cancer?" *Carcinogenesis* 17 no. 3 (1996): 515-523.
       59. doi: 10.1093/carcin/17.3.515.
25.   Jakszyn, P., Gonzalez, C.A. "Nitrosamine and Related Food Intake and Gastric and Oesophageal Cancer Risk: A Systematic Review of the Epidemiological Evidence." *World Journal of Gastroenterology* 12 no. 27 (2006): 4296-4303.
       60. doi: 10.3748/wjg.v12.i27.4296.
26.   Bondonno, C.P., Croft, K.D., Hodgson, J.M. "Dietary Nitrate, Nitric Oxide, and Cardiovascular Health." *Critical Reviews in Food Science and Nutrition* 56 no. 12 (2016): 2036-2052. doi: 10.1080/10408398.2013.811212.
27.   Rostkowska, K., et al. "Formation and Metabolism of Nitrosamines." *Journal of Environmental Studies* 7 no. 6 (1998): 321-325.
28.   Tannenbaum, S.R., Wishnok, J.S., Leaf, C.D. "Inhibition of Nitrosamine Formation by Ascorbic Acid." *The American Journal of Clinical Nutrition* 53 no. 1 (1991): 247S-250S.
29.   International Agency for Research on Cancer. "Press Release No. 240." World Health Organization, October 26, 2015.
30.   Reardon, S. "Food Preservatives Linked to Obesity and Gut Disease." *Nature*, last modified February 25, 2015. doi: 10.1038/nature.2015.16984.
31.   Lan, Z., Yang, W.X. "Nanoparticles and Spermatogenesis: How do Nanoparticles Affect Spermatogenesis and Penetrate the Blood-Testis Barrier." *Nanomedicine* 7 no. 4 (2012). Accessed July 13, 2017. doi: 10.2217/nnm.12.20.
32.   Lockman, P.R., et al. "Nanoparticle Surface Charges Alter Blood-Brain Barrier Integrity and Permeability." *Journal of Drug Targeting* 12 nos. 9-10 (2004): 635-641. doi: 10.1080/10611860400015936.
33.   Lee, J.H., et al. "Biopersistence of Silver Nanoparticles in Tissues from Sprague-Dawley Rats." *Particle and Fibre Toxicology* 10 no. 36 (2013). Accessed July 13, 2017. doi: 10.1186/1743-8977-10-36.
34.   Thakur, M., et al. "Histopathological and Ultra Structural Effects of Nanoparticles on Rat Testis Following 90 Days (Chronic Study) of Repeated Oral Administration." *Journal of Nanobiotechnology* 12 no. 42, (2014). Accessed July 13, 2017.
       61. doi: 10.1186/s12951-014-0042-8.

Chapter 5 – Food Preparation and Packaging

1.   Bassioni, G., et al. "Risk Assessment of Using Aluminum Foil in Food Preparation." *International Journal of Electrochemical Science* 7 (2012): 4498–4509.
2.   Post, G.B., Cohn, P.D., Cooper, K.R. "Perfluorooctanoic Acid (PFOA), An Emerging Drinking Water Contaminant: A Critical Review of Recent Literature." *Environmental Research* 116 (2012): 93–117.

3. Steenland, K., Zhao, L., Winquist, A. "A Cohort Incidence Study of Workers Exposed to Perfluorooctanoic Acid (PFOA)." *Occupational and Environmental Medicine* 72 (2015): 373–380.

4. Barry, V., Winquist, A., Steenland, K. "Perfluorooctanoic Acid (PFOA) Exposures and Incident Cancers Among Adults Living Near a Chemical Plant." *Environmental Health Perspectives* 121 (2013): 1313–1318.

5. Sakr, C.J., et al. "Longitudinal Study of Serum Lipids and Liver Enzymes in Workers with Occupational Exposure to Ammonium Perfluorooctanoate." *Journal of Occupational and Environmental Medicine* 49 no. 8 (2007): 872–879.

6. Melzer, D., et al. "Association Between Serum Perfluoroctanoic Acid (PFOA) and Thyroid Disease in the NHANES Study." *Environmental Health Perspectives* 118 (2010): 686–692.

7. Calafat, A.M., et al. "Serum Concentrations of 11 Polyfluoroalkyl Compounds in the U.S. Population: Data from the National Health and Nutrition Examination Survey (NHANES)." *Environmental Science & Technology* 41 (2007): 2237–2242.

8. Wells, R.E. "Fatal Toxicosis in Pet Birds Caused by an Overheated Cooking Pan Lined with Polytetrafluoroethylene." *Journal of the American Veterinary Medical Association* 182 (1983): 1248–1250.

9. Shuster, K.A., Brock, K.L., Cysko, R.C., et al. "Polytetrafluoroethylene toxicosis in recently hatched chickens (*Gallus domesticus*)." *Comparative Medicine.* 62, no. 1 (Feb 2012): 49–52.

10. Stoltz, J.H., Galey, F., Johnson, B. "Sudden Death in Ten Psittacine Birds Associated with the Operation of a Self-Cleaning Oven." *Veterinary and Human Toxicology* 34 no. 5 (1992): 420–421.

11. Blandford, T.B., et al. "A Case of Polytetrafluoroethylene Poisoning in Cockatiels Accompanied by Polymer Fume Fever in the Owner." *Veterinary Record* 96 (1975): 175–178.

12. Wang, Z., et al. "Chronic Exposure to Aluminum and Risk of Alzheimer's Disease: A Meta-Analysis." *Neuroscience Letters* 610 (Jan 1, 2016): 200–206.

13. Lukiw, W.J., Kruck, T.P., McLachlan, D.R. "Alterations in Human Linker Histone-DNA Binding in the Presence of Aluminum Salts in Vitro and in Alzheimer's Disease." *Neurotoxicology* 8 (1987): 291–301. PMID:3601241.

14. Walton, J.R. "An Aluminum-Based Rat Model for Alzheimer's Disease Exhibits Oxidative Damage, Inhibition of Pp2A Activity, Hyperphosphorylated Tau, and Granulovacuolar Degeneration." *Journal of Inorganic Biochemistry* 101 no. 9 (2007): 1275–1284.

15. Darbre, P.D. "Aluminum, Antiperspirants and Breast Cancer." *Journal of Inorganic Biochemistry* 99 (2005): 1912–1919.

16. Wong, W.W.K., et al. "Dietary Exposure to Aluminum of the Hong Kong Population." *Food Additives & Contaminants: Part A* 27 (2010): 457–463. doi: 10.1080/19440040903490112.

17. Arnich, N., et al. "Dietary Exposure to Trace Elements and Health Risk Assessment in the 2nd French Total Diet Study." *Food and Chemical Toxicology* 50 (2012): 2432–2449.

18.   Saiyed, S.M., Yokel, R.A. "Aluminum Content of Some Foods and Food Products in the USA, with Aluminum Food Additives." *Food Additives & Contaminants* 22 no. 3 (2005): 234–244.

19.   Yang, M., et al. "Dietary Exposure to Aluminum and Health Risk Assessment in the Residents of Shenzhen, China." *PLOS ONE* 9 no. 3 (2014): e89715.

20.   Gramiccioni, L., et al. "Aluminum Levels in Italian Diets and in Selected Foods from Aluminum Utensils." *Food Additives & Contaminants* 13 no. 7 (1996): 767–774.

21.   Ashish, B., Neeti, K., Himanshu, K. "Copper Toxicity: A Comprehensive Study." *Research Journal of Recent Sciences* 2 (2013): 58–67. http://www.isca.in/rjrs/archive/special_issue2012/12.ISCA-ISC-2012-4CS-93.pdf.

22.   Bucossi, S., et al. "Copper in Alzheimer's Disease: A Meta-Analysis of Serum, Plasma, and Cerebrospinal Fluid Studies." *Journal of Alzheimer's Disease* 24 no. 1 (2010): 175–185.

23.   Kamerud, K.L., Hobbie, K.A., Anderson, K.A. "Stainless Steel Leaches Nickel and Chromium into Foods During Cooking." *Journal of Agricultural and Food Chemistry* 61 no. 39 (2013): 9495–9501. http://www.ncbi.nlm.nih.gov/pmc/articles/PMC4284091/.

24.   Zirwas, M.J., Molenda, M.A. "Dietary Nickel as a Cause of Systemic Contact Dermatitis." *The Journal of Clinical and Aesthetic Dermatology* 2 (2009): 39–43. PMCID: PMC2923958.

25.   Abou-Arab, A.K. "Release of Lead from Glaze-Ceramicware into Foods Cooked by Open Flame and Microwave." *Food Chemistry* 73 no. 2 (2001): 163–168. http://www.sciencedirect.com/science/article/pii/S030881460000256 9.

26.   Gould, J.H., et. al. "Hot Leaching of Ceramic and Enameled Ware: A Collaborative Study." *Journal-Association of Official Analytical Chemists* 66 no. 3 (1983). http://www.ncbi.nlm.nih.gov/pubmed/6863183.

27.   Rapaport, M.J., Vinnik, C., Zarem, H. "Injectable Silicone: Cause of Facial Nodules, Cellulitis, Ulceration, and Migration." *Aesthetic Plastic Surgery* 20 no. 3 (1996): 267–276. http://link.springer.com/article/10.1007/s002669900032

28.   McLaughlin, J.K., et.al. "The Safety of Silicone Gel-Filled Breast Implants: A Review of the Epidemiologic Evidence." *Annals of Plastic Surgery* 59 no. 5 (2007): 569–580. http://journals.lww.com/annalsplasticsurgery/Abstract/2007/11000/T he_ Safety_of_Silicone_Gel_Filled_Breast_Implants_.18.aspx.

29.   Vadivambal, R., Jayas, D.S., "Non-Uniform Temperature Distribution During Microwave Heating of Food Materials – A Review." *Food and Bioprocess Technology* 3 no. 2 (2010): 161–171. http://link.springer.com/article/10.1007/s11947-008-0136-0.

30.   Cross, G.A., Fung, D.Y.C., Decareau, R.V. "The Effect of Microwaves on Nutrient Value of Foods." *CRC Critical Reviews in Food Science and Nutrition* 16 no. 4 (1982). http://www.tandfonline.com/doi/abs/10.1080/10408398209527340?s rc=recsys.

31. López-Berenguer, C., et al. "Effects of Microwave Cooking Conditions on Bioactive Compounds Present in Broccoli Inflorescences." *Journal of Agricultural and Food Chemistry* 55 no. 24 (2007): 10001–10007. doi: 10.1021/jf071680t.

32. Valentine, T. "Microwave Tragedy." *Acres USA* (April 1994): 6.

33. De Pomerai, D.I., et al. "Microwave Radiation Can Alter Protein Conformation Without Bulk Heating." *FEBS Letters* 543 nos. 1–3 (2003): 93–97. http://onlinelibrary.wiley.com/doi/10.1016/S0014-5793(03)00413-7/full.

34. Latini, G., Verrotti, A., De Felice, C. "Di-2-Ethylhexyl Phthalate and Endocrine Disruption: A Review." *Current Drug Targets – Immune, Endocrine & Metabolic Disorders* 4 no. 1 (2004): 37–40.

35. Callesen, M., et al. "Phthalate Metabolites in Urine and Asthma, Allergic Rhinoconjunctivitis and Atopic Dermatitis in Preschool Children." *International Journal of Hygiene and Environmental Health* 217 no. 6 (2014): 645-652. doi: 10.1016/j.ijheh.2013.12.001.

36. Shibata, E., et al. "Exposure to House Dust Phthalates in Relation to Asthma and Allergies in Both Children and Adults." *Science of the Total Environment* nos. 485-486 (2014): 153–163. http://hdl.handle.net/2115/55288.

37. Wang, C., et al. "The Classic EDCs, Phthalate Esters and Organochlorines, in Relation to Abnormal Sperm Quality: A Systematic Review with Meta-Analysis." *International Journal of Scientific Reports* 6 (2016): 19982. http://www.ncbi.nlm.nih.gov/pmc/articles/PMC4726156/.

38. Rochester, J.F., Bolden, A.L. "Bisphenol S and F: A Systematic Review and Comparison of the Hormonal Activity of Bisphenol A Substitutes." *Environmental Health Perspectives* 123 no. 7 (2015). doi: 10.1289/ehp.1408989. http://ehp.niehs.nih.gov/1408989/.

39. Liao, C., et al. "Bisphenol S in Urine from the United States and Seven Asian Countries: Occurrence and Human Exposures." *Environmental Science & Technology* 46 no. 12 (2012): 6860–6866. doi: 10.1021/es301334j.

40. Mead, M.N. "CADMIUM CONFUSION: Do Consumers Need Protection?" *Environmental Health Perspectives* 118 no. 12 (2010): A528–A534. 62.doi: 10.1289/ehp.118-a528.

41. Pritchard, J. "Cadmium, Lead Found in Drinking Glasses." Last modified November 22, 2010, http://phys.org/news/2010-11-cadmium-glasses.html.

Chapter 6 – Home Cleaning

1. Bloomfield, S.F., et al. "Time to Abandon the Hygiene Hypothesis: New Perspectives on Allergic Disease, the Human Microbiome, Infectious Disease Prevention and the Role of Targeted Hygiene." *Perspectives in Public Health* 136 no. 4 (2016): 213-224. doi: 10.1177/1757913916650225.

2. Lehtimaki, J., et al. "Patterns in the Skin Microbiota Differ in Children and Teenagers Between Rural and Urban Environments." *Scientific*

Reports 7 (2017): Article number 45651. Accessed July 15, 2017. doi: 10.1038/srep45651.

3.   Jeon, Y.S., Chun, J., Kim, B.S. "Identification of Household Bacterial Community and Analysis of Species Shared with Human Microbiome." *Current Microbiology* 67 no. 5 (2013): 557-563. doi: 10.1007/s00284-013-0401-y.

4.   Strachan, D.P. "Hay Fever, Hygiene, and Household Size." *British Medical Journal* 299 no. 6710 (1989): 1259-1260. PMCID: PMC1838109.

5.   De Coster, S., van Larebeke, N. "Endocrine-Disrupting Chemicals: Associated Disorders and Mechanisms of Action." *Journal of Environmental and Public Health* (2012), Article ID 713696. 52 pages. doi: 10.1155/2012/713696.

6.   Bello, A., et al. "Characterization of Occupational Exposures to Cleaning Products Used for Common Cleaning Tasks - a Pilot Study of Hospital Cleaners." *Environmental Health* 8 no. 11 (2009). Accessed July 15, 2017.
     63. doi: 10.1186/1476-069X-8-11.

7.   Casa, L., et al. "Domestic Use of Bleach and Infections in Children: A Multicentre Cross-Sectional Study." *Occupational & Environmental Medicine* (April 2, 2015). Accessed July 15, 2017. doi: 10.1136/oemed-2014-102701.

8.   Zock, J.P., Vizcaya, D., Le Moual, N. "Update on Asthma and Cleaners." *Current Opinions in Allergy and clinical Immunology* 10 no. 2 (2010): 114-120.
     64. doi: 10.1097/ACI.0b013e32833733fe.

9.   Budama, L., et al. "A New Strategy for Producing Antibacterial Textile Surfaces Using Silver Nanoparticles." *Chemical Engineering Journal* 228 (2013): 489-495. doi: 10.1016/j.cej.2013.05.018.

10. Geranio, L, Heuberger, M., Nowack, B. "The Behavior of Silver Nanotextiles During Washing." *Environmental Science and Technology* 43 no. 21 (2009): 8113-8118. doi: 10.1021/es9018332.

11. U.S. Food & Drug Administration. "Antibacterial Soap? You Can Skip it — Use Plain Soap and Water." Last modified September 2, 2016. Accessed July 16, 2017. https://www.fda.gov/ForConsumers/ConsumerUpdates/ucm378393. htm.

12. Dann, A.B., Hontela, A. "Triclosan: Environmental Exposure, Toxicity and Mechanisms of Action." *Journal of Applied Toxicology* 31 no. 4 (2011): 285-311. doi: 10.1002/jat.1660.

13. Gaulke, C.A., et al. "Triclosan Exposure is Associated with Rapid Restructuring of the Microbiome in Adult Zebrafish." *PLOS ONE* 11 no. 5 (2016): e0154632.
     65. doi: 10.1371/journal.pone.0154632.

14. Barker, J., Jones, M.V. "The Potential Spread of Infection Caused by Aerosol Contamination of Surfaces After Flushing a Domestic Toilet." *Journal of Applied Microbiology* 99 no. 2 (2005): 339-347.

15. Carson, C.F., Hammer, K.A., Riley, T.V. "*Melaleuca alternifolia* (Tea Tree) Oil: a Review of Antimicrobial and Other Medicinal Properties." *Clinical Microbiology Reviews* 19 no. 1 (2006): 50-62. doi: 10.1128/CMR.19.1.50-62.2006.

16.   Rutala, W.A., et al. "Stability and Bactericidal Activity of Chlorine
       Solutions." *Infection Control & Hospital Epidemiology* 19 no. 5
       (1998): 323-327.
       66. PMID: 9613692.
17.   Grice, E.A., Segre, J.A. "The Skin Microbiome." *National Review of
       Microbiology* 9 no. 4 (2011): 244-253. doi: 10.1038/nrmicro2537.
18.   Baldry, M.G.C. "The Bactericidal, Fungicidal and Sporicidal
       Properties of Hydrogen Peroxide and Peracetic Acid." *Journal of
       Applied Microbiology* 54 no. 3 (1983): 417-423. doi: 10.1111/j.1365-
       2672.1983.tb02637.x.
19.   Anderson, S.E., Meade, B.J. "Potential Health Effects Associated
       with Dermal Exposure to Occupational Chemicals." *Environmental
       Health Insights* 8 no. 1 (2014): 51-62. doi: 10.4137/EHI.S15258.
20.   Peck, B., et al. "Spectrum of Sodium Hypochlorite Toxicity in Man -
       Also a Concern for Nephrologists." Clinical Kidney Journal 4 no. 4
       2(011): 231-235.
       67. doi: 10.1093/ndtplus/sfr053.
21.   Quinn, M.M., Henneberger, P.K. "Cleaning and Disinfecting
       Environmental Surfaces in Health Care: Toward an Integrated
       Framework for Infection and Occupational Illness Prevention."
       Control 43 no. 5 (2015): 424-434.
       68. doi: 10.1016/j.ajic.2015.01.029.
22.   Gosselin, R.E., Smith, R.P., Hodge, H.C. "Clinical Toxicology of
       Commercial Products. 5th ed." Baltimore: Williams and Wilkins
       (1984): III-22.
23.   "FAQ – Why did Pine-Sol change the original formula?" Pine-Sol
       (Official page via Facebook). Accessed August 26, 2016.
24.   Wolkoff, P., Nielsen, G.D. "Effects by Inhalation of Abundant
       Fragrances in Indoor Air - An Overview." *Environment International*
       101 (2017): 96-107.
       69. doi: 10.1016/j.envint.2017.01.013.
25.   Gerster, F.M., et al. "Hazardous Substances in Frequently Used
       Professional Cleaning Products." *International Journal of
       Occupational and Environmental Health* 20 no. 1 (2014): 46-60. doi:
       10.1179/2049396713Y.0000000052.
26.   Kapuci, M., et al. "Determination of Cytotoxic and Genotoxic Effects
       of Nappthalene, 1-naphthol and 2-naphthol on Human Lymphocyte
       culture." *Toxicology and Industrial Health* 30 no. 1, (2014): 82-89.
       doi:10.1177/0748233712451772.
27.   Green, T., et al. "Perchloroethylene-Induced Rat Kidney Tumors: An
       Investigation of the Mechanisms Involved and their Relevance to
       Humans." *Toxicology and Applied Pharmacology* 103 no. 1, (1990):
       77-89.
       70. doi: 10.1016/0041-008X(90)90264-U.
28.   Lieder, P.H., et al. "A Two-Generation Oral Gavage Reproduction
       Study with Potassium Perfuorobutanesulfonate (K$^+$PFBS) in
       Sprague Dawley Rats." *Toxicology* 259 nos. 1-2 (2009): 33-45. doi:
       10.1016/j.tox.2009.01.027.
29.   Olsen, G.W., et al. "A Comparison of the Pharmacokinetics of
       Perfluorobutanesulfonate (PFBS) in Rats, Monkeys, and Humans."

Toxicology 256 nos. 1-2 (2009): 65-74. doi:
10.1016/j.tox.2008.11.008.

30.   Aiso, S., et al. "Carcinogenicity and Chronic Toxicity in Mice and
       Rats Exposed by Inhalation to Para-Dichlorobenzene for Two
       Years." *Journal of Veterinary Medical Science* 67 (2005): 1019-
       1029. PMID: 16276058.

31.   U.S. Department of Health and Human Services Data Bank.
       Bethesda, MD: National Toxicology Information Program, National
       Library of Medicine, 1993.

32.   Agency for Toxic Substances and Disease Registry (ATSDR).
       "Toxicological Profile for 1,4-Dichlorobenzene (Update)." Atlanta:
       Public Health Service, U.S. Department of Health and Human
       Services, 1998.

33.   Elliott, L., et al. "Volatile Organic Compounds and Pulmonary
       Function in the Third National Health and Nutrition Examination
       Survey, 1988-1994." *Environmental Health Perspectives* 114 no. 8
       (2006): 1210-1214. PMCID: PMC1551996.

34.   Cheong R., et al. "Mothball Withdrawal Encephalopathy: Case
       Report and Review of Paradichlorobenzene Neurotoxicity."
       Substance Abuse 27 no. 4 (2006): 63-67. PMID: 17347127.

35.   Cohen, A., Janssen, S., Solomon, G. "Clearing the Air: Hidden
       Hazards of Air Fresheners." *National Resources Defense Council*
       (September 2007.)
       71. https://www.researchgate.net/publication/262872839_Clearing_t
       he_Air_Hidden_Hazards_of_Air_Fresheners.

36.   Caress, S.M., Steinemann, A.C. "Prevalence of Fragrance
       Sensitivity in the American Population." *Journal of Environmental
       Health* 71 no. 7 (2009): 46-50. PMID: 19326669.

37.   Mohagheghzadeh, A., et al. "Medicinal Smokes." *Journal of
       Ethnopharmacology* 108 no. 2 (2006): 161-184. PMID: 17030480.

Chapter 7 – Personal Care Products

1.   Yaemsiri S., et al. "Growth Rate of Human Fingernails and Toenails
       in Healthy American Young Adults." *Journal of the European
       Academy of Dermatology and Venereology* 24 no. 4 (2010): 420-
       423. doi: 10.1111/j.1468-3083.2009.03426.x.

2.   Funt, D., Pavicic, T. "Dermal Fillers in Aesthetics: An Overview of
       Adverse Events and Treatment Approaches." *Clinical, Cosmetic and
       Investigational Dermatology* 6 (2013): 295-316. doi:
       10.2147/CCID.S50546.

3.   Borumand, M., Sibilla, S. "Effects of a Nutritional Supplement
       Containing Collagen Peptides on Skin Elasticity, Hydration and
       Wrinkles." *Journal of Medical Nutrition & Nutraceuticals* 4 no. 1
       (2015): 47-53. doi: 10.4103/2278-019X.146161.

4.   Grice, E.A., Segre J.A. "The Skin Microbiome." *National Reviews of
       Microbiology* 9 no. 4 (2011): 244-253. doi: 10.1038/nrmicro2537.

5.   Cogen, A.L., Nizet, V., Gallo, R.L. "Skin Microbiota: A Source of
       Disease or Defence?" *British Journal of Dermatology* 158 no. 3
       (2008): 442-455.
       72. doi: 10.1111/j.1365-2133.2008.08437.x.

6. Allhorn, M., et al. "A Novel Enzyme with Antioxidant Capacity Produced by the Ubiquitous Skin Colonizer *Propionibacterium acnes*." *Scientific Reports* 6 (2016): Article number: 36412. Accessed July 18, 2017. doi: 10.1038/srep36412.

7. Grice, E.A., et al. "Topographical and Temporal Diversity of the Human Skin Microbiome." *Science* 324 no. 5931 (2009): 1190-1192. 73. doi: 10.1126/science.1171700.

8. Biniek, K., Levi, K., Dauskardt, R.H. "Solar UV Radiation Reduces the Barrier Function of Human Skin." *Proceedings of the National Academy of Sciences of the United States of America* 109 no. 42 (2012): 17111-17116. Accessed July 18, 2017. doi: 10.1073/pnas.1206851109.

9. Baroli, B. "Penetration of Nanoparticles and Nanomaterials in the Skin: Fiction or Reality?" *Journal of Pharmaceutical Sciences* 99 no. 1 (2010): 21-50. 74. doi: 10.1002/jps.21817.

10. Wallen-Russell, C., Wallen-Russell, S. "Meta Analysis of Skin Microbiome: New Link Between Skin Microbiota Diversity and Skin Health with Proposal to Use This as a Future Mechanism to Determine Whether Cosmetic Products Damage the Skin." *Cosmetics* 4 no. 14 (2017): 1-19. Accessed July 18, 2017. 75. doi: 10.3390/cosmetics4020014.

11. Cramer, D.W., et al. "The Association Between Talc Use and Ovarian Cancer: A Retrospective Case-Control Study in Two US States." *Epidemiology* 27 no. 3, (2016): 334-346. doi: 10.1097/EDE.0000000000000434.

12. James-Todd, T., et al. "Childhood Hair Product Use and Earlier Age at Menarche in a Racially Diverse Study Population: A Pilot Study." *Annals of Epidemiology* 21 no. 6 (2011): 461-465. doi: 10.1016/j.annepidem.2011.01.009.

13. Apter, D., Vihko, R. "Early Menarche, A Risk Factor for Breast Cancer, Indicates Early Onset of Ovulatory Cycles." *Journal of Clinical Endocrinology & Metabolism* 57 no. 1 (1983): 82-86. doi: 10.1210/jcem-57-1-82.

14. Stiel, L., et al. "A Review of Hair Product Use on Breast Cancer Risk in African American Women." *Cancer Medicine* 5 no. 3, (2016): 597-604. 76. doi: 10.1002/cam4.613.

15. Hepp, N.M. "Determination of Total Lead in 400 Lipsticks on the U.S. Market Using a Validated Microwave-Assisted Digestion Inductively Coupled Plasma-Mass Spectrometric Method." *Journal of Cosmetic Science* 63 (2012): 159-176.

16. Zulaikha, S., Syed Ismail, S., Praveena, S. "Hazardous Ingredients in Cosmetics and Personal Care Products and Health Concern: A Review." *Public Health Research* no. 1 (2015): 7-15. doi: 10.5923/j.phr.20150501.02.

17. "Heavy Metal Hazard, the Health Risks of Hidden Heavy Metals in Face Makeup." *Environmental Defence Canada* (2011).

18. Volpe, M.G., et al. "Determination and Assessments of Selected Heavy Metals in Eye Shadow Cosmetics from China, Italy, and USA." *Microchemical Journal* 101 (2012): 65-69.

19.   Johansen, J.D. "Fragrance Contact Allergy: A Clinical Review."
      American Journal of Clinical Dermatology 4 no. 11 (2003): 789-798.
      PMID: 14572300.
20.   Latha, M.S., et al. "Sunscreening Agents." *The Journal of Clinical
      and Aesthetic Dermatology* 6 no. 1 (2013): 16-26. PMCID:
      PMC3543289.
21.   Department of Health and Human Services, Food and Drug
      Administration. "Sunscreen Drug Products for Over-the-Counter
      Human Use; Final Rules and Proposed Rules." *Federal Register*,
      Part IV. 21 CFR Parts 201, 310, and 352. June 17, 2011. Accessed
      November 15, 2012.
      77. http://www.gpo.gov/fdsys/pkg/FR-2011-06-17/pdf/2011-
      14766.pdf.
22.   Green, A., et al. "Daily Sunscreen Application and Betacarotene
      Supplementation in Prevention of Basal-Cell and Squamous-Cell
      Carcinomas of the Skin: A Randomised Controlled Trial." *The
      Lancet* 354 no. 9180 (1999): 723-729.
      78. doi: 10.1016/S0140-6736(98)12168-2.
23.   Dennis, L.K., et al. "Sunburns and Risk of Cutaneous Melanoma,
      Does Age Matter: A Comprehensive Meta-Analysis." *Annals of
      Epidemiology* 18 no. 8 (2008): 614-627. doi:
      10.1016/j.annepidem.2008.04.006.
24.   Krause, M., et al. "Sunscreens: Are They Beneficial for Health? An
      Overview of Endocrine Disrupting Properties of UV-Filters."
      International Journal of Andrology 35 no. 3 (2012): 424-436. doi:
      10.1111/j.1365-2605.2012.01280.x.

Chapter 8 – Sound

1.   Galambos, R., Hecox, K.E. "Clinical Applications of the Auditory
      Brain Stem Response." *Otolaryngologic Clinics of North America* 11
      no. 3 (1978): 709-722. PMID: 733255.
2.   Kotsovolis, G., Komninos, G. "Awareness During Anesthesia: How
      Sure Can We be that the Patient is Sleeping Indeed?" *Hippokratia*
      13 no. 2 (2009): 83-89.
      79. PMCID: PMC2683150.
3.   Klatte, M., Bergstrom, K., Lachmann, T. "Does Noise Affect
      Learning? A Short Review on Noise Effects on Cognitive
      Performance in Children." *Frontiers in Psychology* 4 (2013): 578.
      doi: 10.3389/fpsyg.2013.00578.
4.   Lee, O.K., et al. "Music and its Effect on the Physiological
      Responses and Anxiety Levels of Patients Receiving Mechanical
      Ventilation: A Pilot Study." *Journal of Clinical Nursing* 14 no. 5
      (2005): 609-620. doi: 10.1111/j.1365-2702.2004.01103.x.
5.   Juslin, P.N., Vastfjall, D. "Emotional Responses to Music: The Need
      to Consider Underlying Mechanisms." The *Behavioral and Brain
      Sciences* 31 no. 5 (2008): 559-575. doi:
      10.1017/S0140525X08005293.
6.   Strogatz, S.H., Stewart, I. "Coupled Oscillators and Biological
      Synchronization." *Scientific American* 269 no. 6 (1993): 102-109.
      PMID: 8266056.

7. Kelly, J.R. "Entrainment in Individual and Group Behavior." In *The Social Psychology of Time: New Perspectives*, edited by J.E. McGrath, 89-112. Thousand Oaks, CA: Sage, 1988.

8. Weller, A., Weller, L. "Menstrual Synchrony Between Mothers and Daughters and Between Roommates." *Physiology & Behavior* 53 no. 5 (1993): 943-949.
    80. doi: 10.1016/0031-9384(93)90273-I.

9. Watanabe, T., Okubo, M. "Evaluation of the Entrainment Between a Speaker's Burst-Pause of Speech and Respiration and a Listener's Respiration in Face-to-Face Communication." *Robot and Human Communication* (1997) RO-MAN '97. Proceedings, 6th IEEE International Workshop.
    81. doi: 10.1109/ROMAN.1997.647018.

10. Bernardi, L, et al. "Dynamic Interactions Between Musical, Cardiovascular, and Cerebral Rhythms in Humans." *Circulation* 119 (2009): 3171-3180.
    82. doi: 10.1161/CIRCULATIONAHA.108.806174.

11. Loewy, J., et al. "The Effects of Music Therapy on Vital Signs, Feeding, and Sleep in Premature Infants." *Pediatrics* 131 (2013): 902-918.
    83. doi: 10.1542/peds.2012-1367.

12. Glass, L. "Synchronization and Rhythmic Processes in Physiology." *Nature* 410 (2001): 277-284. doi: 10.1038/35065745.

13. Kim, D-K., et al. "Dynamic Correlations Between Heart and Brain Rhythm During Autogenic Meditation." *Frontiers in Human Neuroscience* 7 (2013): 414. Accessed July 20, 2017. doi: 10.3389/fnhum.2013.00414.

14. Campbell, D. *The Mozart Effect.* New York: Avon Books, 1997.

15. Jenkins, J.S. "The Mozart Effect." *Journal of the Royal Society of Medicine* 94 no. 4 (2001): 170-172. PMCID: PMC1281386.

16. Graziano, A.B., Peterson, M., Shaw, G.L. "Enhanced Learning of Proportional Math through Music Training and Spatial-Temporal Training." *Neurological Research* 21 no. 2 (1999): 139-152.

17. Rideout B.E., Dougherty, S., Wernert L. "Effect of Music on Spatial Performance: A Test of Generality." *Perceptual and Motor Skills Research Exchange* 86 (1998): 512-514. doi: 10.2466/pms.1998.86.2.512.

18. Lin, F.R., Niparko, J.K., Ferrucci, L. "Hearing Loss Prevalence in the United States." *Archives of Internal Medicine* 171 no. 20 (2011): 1851-1852.
    84. doi: 10.1001/archinternmed.2011.506.

19. Portnuff, C.D.F. "Reducing the Risk of Music-Induced Hearing Loss from Overuse of Portable Listening Devices: Understanding the Problems and Establishing Strategies for Improving Awareness in Adolescents." *Adolescent Health, Medicine and Therapeutics* 7 (2016): 27-35. doi: 10.2147/AHMT.S74103.

20. Rabinowitz, P.M. "Noise-Induced Hearing Loss." *American Family Physician* 61 no. 9 (2000): 2749-2756, 2759-2760. PMID: 10821155.

21.   Jahrsdoefer, R. "The Effects of Impulse Noise on the Eardrum and Middle Ear." *Otolaryngolocial Clinics of North America* 12 no. 3 (1979): 515-520. PMID: 471499.

22.   Wong, A.C.Y., Ryan, A.F. "Mechanisms of Sensorineural Cell Damage, Death and Survival in the Cochlea." *Frontiers in Aging Neuroscience* 7 (2015): 58. Accessed July 20, 2017. doi: 10.3389/fnagi.2015.00058.

23.   Burnett, J., et al. "Warning: Exercise May Damage Your Hearing." *Education* 3 no. 3 (2013): 157-160. doi: 10.5923/j.edu.20130303.03.

24.   Vogel, I., et al. "MP3 Players and Hearing Loss: Adolescent Perceptions of Loud Music and Hearing Conversation." *Journal of Pediatrics* 152 (2008): 400-404.
       85. doi: 10.1016/j.jpeds.2007.07.009.

25.   Curhan, S.G., et al. "Analgesic Use and the Risk of Hearing Loss in Men." *American Journal of Medicine* 123 no. 3 (2010): 231-237.
       86. doi: 10.1016/j.amjmed.2009.08.006.

26.   Huang, M.Y., Schacht, J. "Drug-Induced Ototoxicity." *Medical Toxicology and Adverse Drug Experience* 4 no. 6 (1989): 452-467.

27.   Pascuan, C.G., et al. "Immune Alterations Induced by Chronic Noise Exposure: Comparison with Restraint Stress in BALB/c and C57Bl/6 Mice." *Journal of Immunotoxicology* 11 no. 1 (2014): 78-83. doi: 10.3109/1547691X.2013.800171.

28.   Ristovska, G., Laszio, H.E., Hansell, A.L. "Reproductive Outcomes Associated with Noise Exposure - A Systematic Review of the Literature." *International Journal of Environmental Research and Public Health* 11 no. 8 (2014): 7931-7952.
       87. doi: 10.3390/ijerph110807931.

29.   Basner, M., et al. "Auditory and Non-Auditory Effects of Noise on Health." *The Lancet* 383 no. 9925 (2014): 1325-1332. doi: 10.1016/S0140-6736(13)61613-X.

30.   Ising, H., Braun, C. "Acute and Chronic Endocrine Effects of Noise: Review of the Research Conducted at the Institute for Water, Soil and Air Hygiene." *Noise & Health* 2 no. 7 (2000): 7-24.

31.   Leventhall, G., Pelmear, P., Benton, S. "A Review of Published Research on Low Frequency Noise and its Effects." *Westminster Research,* 2003. Accessed July 20, 2017. http://westminsterresearch.wmin.ac.uk.

32.   Iwanga, M., Moroki, Y. "Subjective and Physiological Responses to Music Stimuli Controlled over Activity and Preference." *Journal of Music Therapy* 36 no. 1 (1999): 26-38. doi: 10.1093/jmt/36.1.26.

33.   Leeds, J. "The Power of Sound: How to Manage Your Personal Soundscape for a Vital, Productive & Healthy Life." Rochester, VT: Healing Arts Press, 2001.

Chapter 9 – EMF

1.   Wiltschko, W., Wiltschko, R. "Magnetic Orientation and Magnetoreception in Birds and Other Animals." *Journal of Comparative Physiology A* 191 no. 8 (2005): 675-693. doi: 10.1007/s00359-005-0627-7.

2. Nakagawa, K. "Magnetic Deficiency Syndrome and Magnetic Treatment." Translated article from *Japan Medical Journal* 2745 (1976). Accessed July 21, 2017. http://4data.ca/ottawa/archive/health/biomagnetic.html.

3. Rochalska, M. "The Influence of Electromagnetic Fields on Flora and Fauna." *Medycyna Pracy* 60 no. 1 (2009): 43-50. PMID: 19603696.

4. Lohmann, K.J., Lohmann, C.M., Putman, N.F. "Magnetic Maps in Animals: Nature's GPS." *Journal of Experimental Biology* 210 (2007): 3697-3705. 88. doi: 10.1242/jeb.001313.

5. Ross, C.L. "The Effect of Low-Frequency Electromagnetic Field on Human Bone Marrow Stem/Progenitor Cell Differentiation." *Stem Cell Research* 15 no. 1 (2015): 96-108. doi: 10.1016/j.scr.2015.04.009.

6. Nguyen, T.H.P., et al. "18 GHz Electromagnetic Field Induces Permeability of Gram-Positive Cocci." *Scientific Reports* 5 (2015): 10980. Accessed July 22, 2017. doi: 10.1038/srep10980.

7. Pall, M.L. "Microwave Frequency Electromagnetic Fields (EMFs) Produce Widespread Neuropsychiatric Effects Including Depression." *Journal of Chemical Neuroanatomy* 75 Part B (2016): 43-51. doi: 10.1016/j.jchemneu.2015.08.001.

8. Bawin, S.M., Adey, W.R. "Sensitivity of Calcium Binding in Cerebral Tissue to Weak Environmental Electric Fields Oscillating at Low Frequency." *Proceedings of the National Academy of Sciences of the United States of America* 73 no. 6 (1976): 1999-2003. PMCID: PMC430435.

9. Blackman, D.F., et al. "Effects of ELF Fields on Calcium-Ion Efflux from Brain Tissue in Vitro." *Radiation Research* 92 no. 3 (1982): 510-520.

10. Matthews, E.K. "Calcium and Membrane Permeability." *British Medical Bulletin* 42 no. 4 (1986): 391-397. https://doi.org/10.1093/oxfordjournals.bmb.a072157.

11. Mortavazi, S., et al. "Alterations in TSH and Thyroid Hormones Following Mobile Phone Use." *Oman Medical Journal* 24 no. 4 (2009): 274-278. 89. doi: 10.5001/omj.2009.56.

12. Koyu, A., et al. "Effects of 900 MHz Electomagnetic Field on TSH and Thyroid Hormones in Rats." *Toxicology Letters* 157 no. 3 (2005): 257-262. 90. doi: 10.1016/j.toxlet.2005.03.006.

13. Gorpinchenko, I., et al. "The Influence of Direct Mobile Phone Radiation on Sperm Quality." *Central European Journal of Urology* 67 no. 1 (2014): 65-71. 91. doi: 10.5173/ceju.2014.01.art14.

14. Agarwal, A., et. al. "Effect of Cell Phone Usage on Semen Analysis in Men Attending Infertility Clinic: An Observational Study." *Fertility and Sterility* 89 no. 1 (2008): 124-128. doi: 10.1016/j.fertnstert.2007.01.166.

15. Kliukiene, J., Tynes, T., Andersen, A. "Follow-Up of Radio and Telegraph Operators with Exposure to Electromagnetic Fields and

Risk of Breast Cancer." *European Journal of Cancer Prevention* 12 no 4 (2003): 301-307.
92. doi: 10.1097/01.cej.0000082602.47188.da.

16. Chen, Q., et al. "A Meta-Analysis on the Relationship Between Exposure to ELF-EMFs and the Risk of Female Breast Cancer." *PLOS ONE* 8 no. 7 (2013): e69272. doi: 10.1371/journal.pone.0069272.

17. International Agency for Research on Cancer. "Press Release No. 208 - IARC Classifies Radiofrequency Electromagnetic Fields as Possibly Carcinogenic to Humans." Geneva: World Health Organization, May 31, 2011.

18. Davis, S. "Weak Residential Magnetic Fields Affect Melatonin in Humans." *Microwave News* 17 no. 6. (Nov/Dec 1997). 1,4.

19. Volkow, N.D., et al. "Effects of Cell Phone Radiofrequency Signal Exposure on Brain Glucose Metabolism." *Journal of the American Medical Association* 305 no. 8 (2011): 808-813. doi: 10.1001/jama.2011.186.

20. Santini, R., et al. "Survey Study of People Living in the Vicinity of Cellular Phone Base Stations." *Electromagnetic Biology and Medicine* 22 no. 1 (2003): 41-49.

21. Gomez-Perretta, C., et al. "Subjective Symptoms Related to GSM Radiation from Mobile Phone Base Stations: A Cross-Sectional Study." *British Medical Journal* 3 no. 12 (2013): e003836. doi: 10.1136/bmjopen-2013-003836.

22. Hardell, L., et al. "Vestibular Schwannoma, Tinnitus and Cellular Telephones." *Neuroepidemiology* 22 no. 2 (2003): 124-129. doi: 10.1159/000068745.

23. Frei, P., et al. "Residential Distance to High-Voltage Power Lines and Risk of Neurodegenerative Diseases: A Danish Population-Based Case-Control Study." *American Journal of Epidemiology* 177 no. 9 (2013): 970-978.
93. doi: 10.1093/aje/kws334.

24. Mattson, M.O., Simko, M. "Is There a Relation Between Extremely Low Frequency Magnetic Field Exposure, Inflammation and Neurodegenerative Diseases? A Review of in Vivo and in Vitro Experimental Evidence." *Toxicology* 301 nos. 1-3 (2012): 1-12. doi: 10.1016/j.tox.2012.06.011.

25. "IARC Report to the Union for International Cancer Control (UICC) on the Interphone Study." Geneva: World Health Organization, 2011.

26. Yang, M., et al. "Mobile Phone Use and Glioma Risk: A Systematic Review and Meta-Analysis." *PLOS ONE* 12 no. 5 (2017): e0175136.
94. doi: 10.1371/journal.pone.0175136.

27. Hardell, L., Carlberg, M. "Mobile Phone and Cordless Phone Use and the Risk for Glioma - Analysis of Pooled Case-Control Studies in Sweden, 1997-2003 and 2007-2009." *Pathophysiology* 22 no. 1 (2015): 1-13.
95. doi: 10.1016/j.pathophys.2014.10.001.

28. Kheifets, L. "Pooled Analysis of Recent Studies on Magnetic Fields and Childhood Leukaemia." *British Journal of Cancer* 103 no. 7 (2010): 1128-1135.

96. doi: 10.1038/sj.bjc.6605838.

29. De-Kun, L., et al. "A Population-Based Prospective Cohort Study of Personal Exposure to Magnetic Fields During Pregnancy and the Risk of Miscarriage." *Epidemiology* 13 no.1 (2002): 9-20.

30. Belanger, K., et al. "Spontaneous Abortion and Exposure to Electric Blankets and Heated Water Beds." *Epidemiology* 9 no. 1 (1998): 36-42. PMID: 9430266.

31. Wang, Q., et al. "Residential Exposure to 50 Hz Magnetic Fields and the Association with Miscarriage Risk: A 2-Year Prospective Cohort Study." *PLOS ONE* 8 no. 12 (2013): e82113. doi: 10.1371/journal.pone.0082113.

Chapter 10 – Light

1. Zimecki, M. "The Lunar Cycle: Effects on Human and Animal Behavior and Physiology." *Postepy Higieny I Modycyny Doswiadczalnej* 60 (2006): 1-7. PMID: 16407788.

2. Tosini, G., Ferguson, I., Tsubota, K. "Effects of Blue Light on the Circadian System and Eye Physiology." *Molecular Vision* 22 (2016): 61-72. Accessed July 24, 2017. PMCID: PMC4734149.

3. Bayliss, C.R., Bishop, N.L., Fowler, R.C. "Pineal Gland Calcification and Defective Sense of Direction." *British Medical Journal* 291 no. 6511 (1985): 1758-1759. PMCID: PMC1419179.

4. Premkumar, M., et al. "Circadian Levels of Serum Melatonin and Cortisol in Relation to Changes in Mood, Sleep, and Neurocognitive Performance, Spanning a Year of Residence in Antartica." *Neuroscience Journal* 2013 (2013). Accessed July 24, 2017. doi: 10.1155/2013/254090.

5. Adamsson, M., Laike, T., Morita, T. "Annual Variation in Daily Light Exposure and Circadian Change of Melatonin and Cortisol Concentrations at a Northern Latitude with Large Seasonal Differences in Photoperiod Length." *Journal of Physiological Anthropology* 36 no. 6 (2016). 97. doi: 10.1186/s40101-016-0103-9.

6. Srinivasan, V., et al. "Melatonin, Immune Function and Aging." *Immunity & Ageing* 2 no. 17 (2005). doi: 10.1186/1742-4933-2-17.

7. Li, W., et al. "Melatonin Treatment Induces Apoptosis Through Regulating the Nuclear Factor-KB and Mitogen-Activated Protein Kinase Signaling Pathways in Human Gastric Cancer SGC7901 Cells." *Oncology Letters* 13 no. 4 (2017): 2737-2744. doi: 10.3892/ol.2017.5785.

8. Luboshitzky, R., Lavie, P. "Melatonin and Sex Hormone Interrelationships – A Review." *Journal of Pediatric Endocrinology & Metabolism* 12 no. 3 (1999): 355-362. PMID: 10821215.

9. Korkmaz, A., Rosales-Corral, S., Reiter, R. "Gene Regulation by Melatonin Linked to Epigenetic Phenomena." *Gene* 503 no. 1 (2012): 1-11. 98. doi: 10.1016/j.gene.2012.04.040.

10. Pacchierotti, C., et al. "Melatonin in Psychiatric Disorders: A Review on the Melatonin Involvement in Psychiatry." *Frontiers in*

Neuroendocrinology 22 no. 1 (2001): 18-32. doi: 10.1006/frne.2000.0202.

11.   Gooley, J.J., et al. "Exposure to Room Light Before Bedtime Suppresses Melatonin Onset and Shortens Melatonin Duration in Humans." *Journal of Clinical Endocrinology & Metabolism* 96 no. 3 (2011): E463-E472.
99. doi: 10.1210/jc.2010-2098.

12.   Cajochen, C., et al. "Evening Exposure to a Light-Emitting Diodes (LED)-Backlit Computer Screen Affects Circadian Physiology and Cognitive Performance." *Journal of Applied Physiology* 110 no. 5 (2011): 1432-1438.
100.   doi: 10.1152/japplphysiol.00165.2011.

13.   Higuchi, S., et al. "Influence of Light at Night on Melatonin Suppression in Children." *Journal of Clinical Endocrinology & Metabolism* 99 no. 9 (2014): 3298-3303. doi: 10.1210/jc.2014-1629.

14.   Cajochen, C., Krauchi, K., Wirz-Justice, A. "Role of Melatonin in the Regulation of Human Circadian Rhythms and Sleep." *Journal of Neuroendocrinology* 15 no. 4 (2003): 432-437. doi: 10.1046/j.1365-2826.2003.00989.x.

15.   Stevens, R.G., Rea, M.S. "Light in the Built Environment: Potential Role of Circadian Disruption in Endocrine Disruption and Breast Cancer." *Cancer Causes & Control* 12 no. 3 (2001): 279-287.

16.   Knutsson, A. "Health Disorders of Shift Workers." *Occupational Medicine* 53 no. 2 (2003): 103-108. doi: 10.1093/occmed/kqg048.

17.   Grundy, A., et al. "Increased Risk of Breast Cancer Associated with Long-Term Shift Work in Canada." *Occupational and Environmental Medicine* 70 no. 12 (2013): 831-838.

18.   Pinkerton, L.E., et al. "Breast Cancer Incidence Among Female Flight Attendants: Exposure-Response Analyses." *Scandinavian Journal of Work, Environment & Health* 42 no. 6 (2016): 538-546. doi: 10.5271/sjweh.3586.

19.   Kloog, I., et al. "Does the Modern Urbanized Sleeping Habitat Pose a Breast Cancer Risk?" *Chronobiology International* 28 no. 1 (2011): 76-80.
101.   doi: 10.3109/07420528.2010.531490.

20.   Kloog, I., et al. "Light at Night -Co-Distributes with Incident Breast but not Lung Cancer in the Female Population of Israel." *Chronobiology International* 25 no. 1 (2008): 65-81. doi: 10.1080/07420520801921572.

21.   Reiter, R.J., et al. "Light at Night, Chronodisruption, Melatonin Suppression, and Cancer Risk: A Review." *Critical Reviews in Oncogenesis* 13 no. 4 (2007): 303-328. doi: 10.1615/CritRevOncog.v13.i4.30.

22.   Zeitzer, J.M., et al. "Millisecond Flashes of Light Phase Delay the Human Circadian Clock During Sleep." *Journal of Biological Rhythms* 29 no. 5 (2014): 370-376.
102.   doi: 10.1177/0748730414546532.

23.   Chojnacki, C., Blonska, A., Chojnacki, J. "The Effects of Melatonin on Elevated Liver Enzymes During Statin Treatment." *BioMed Research International* 2017 (2017): 3204504. doi: 10.1155/2017/3204504.

24. Pandi-Perumal, S.R., et al. "Melatonin." *The FEBS Journal* 273 no. 13 (2006): 2813-2838. doi: 10.1111/j.1742-4658.2006.05322.x.

25. Rosen, L.N., et al. "Prevalence of Seasonal Affective Disorder at Four Latitudes." *Psychiatry Research* 31 no. 2 (1990): 131-144. PMID: 2326393.

26. Rosenthal, N.E., et al. "Seasonal Affective Disorder: A Description of the Syndrome and Preliminary Findings with Light Therapy." *Archives of General Psychiatry* 41 no. 1 (1984): 72-80. PMID: 6581756.

27. Rosenthal, N.E., et al. "Melatonin in Seasonal Affective Disorder and Phototherapy." *Journal of Neural Transmission Supplement* 21 (1986): 257-267. PMID: 3462335.

28. Papamichael, K., et al. "High Color Rendering Can Enable Better Vision without Requiring More Power." *The Journal of the Illuminating Engineering Society* 12 nos. 1-2 (2016): 27-38. doi: 10.1080/15502724.2015.1004412.

29. Sayre, R.M., Dowdy, J.C., Poh-Fitzpatrick, M. "Dermatological Risk of Indoor Ultraviolet Exposure from Contemporary Lighting Sources." *Photochemistry and Photobiology* 80 no. 1 (2004): 47-51. doi: 10.1562/2004-02-03-RA-074.1.

30. Bloom, E., et al. "Halogen Lamp Phototoxicity." *Dermatology* 193 no. 3 (1996): 207-211. PMID: 8944342.

31. Kondro, W. "Mercury Disposal Sole Health Concern with Fluorescent Lights." *Canadian Medical Association Journal* 177 no. 2 (2007): 136-137.
103. doi: 10.1503/cmaj.070816.

32. Li, Y., Jin, L. "Environmental Release of Mercury from Broken Compact Fluorescent Lamps." *Environmental Engineering Science* 28 no. 10 (2011): 687-691. doi: 10.1089/ees.2011.0027.

33. Johnson, N.C., et al. "Mercury Vapor Release from Broken Compact Fluorescent Lamps and In Situ Capture by New Nanomaterial Sorbents." *Environmental Science & Technology* 42 no. 15 (2008): 5772-5778. doi: 10.1021/es8004392.

34. Mironava, T., et al. "The Effects of UV Emission from Compact Fluorescent Light Exposure on Human Dermal Fibroblasts and Keratinocytes *In Vitro*." *Photochemistry and Photobiology* 88 no. 6 (2012): v1497-1506.
104. doi: 10.1111/j.1751-1097.2012.01192.x.

35. Safari, S., et al. "Ultraviolet Radiation Emissions and Illuminance in Different Brands of Compact Fluorescent Lamps." *International Journal of Photoenergy* 2015 (2015): 6 pages. doi: 10.1155/2015/504674.

36. Fenton, L., Ferguson, J., Moseley, H. "Analysis of Energy Saving Lamps for Use by Photosensitive Individuals." *Photochemical & Photobiological Sciences* 11 no. 8 (2012): 1346-1355. doi: 10.1039/c2pp25035g.

37. Olle, M., Virsile, A. "The Effects of Light Emitting Diode on Greenhouse Plant Growth and Quality." *Agricultural and Food Science* 22 no. 2 (2013): 223-234.

38. Vandewalle, G., et al. "Blue Light Stimulates Cognitive Brain Activity in Visually Blind Individuals." *Journal of Cognitive Neuroscience* 25 no. 12 (2013): 2072-2085. doi: 10.1162/jocn_a_00450.
39. Vandewalle, G., et al. "Spectral Quality of Light Modulates Emotional Brain Responses in Humans." *Proceedings of the National Academy of Sciences of the United States of America* 107 no. 45 (2010): 19549-19554.
     105. doi: 10.1073/pnas.1010180107.

Chapter 11 – Feng Shui

Chapter 12 – Meditation

1. Delui, M.H., et al. "Comparison of Cardiac Rehabilitation Programs Combined with Relaxation and Meditation Techniques on Reduction of Depression and Anxiety of Cardiovascular Patients." The *Open Cardiovascular Medical Journal* 18 no. 7 (2013): 99-103. doi: 10.2174/1874192401307010099.
2. Morgan, Nani, et al. "The Effects of Mind-Body Therapies on the Immune System: Meta-Analysis *PLOS ONE* (2014). Accessed July 26, 2017.
    106. doi: 10.1371/journal.pone.0100903.
3. Govindaraj, R., Karmani, S., Varambally, S. "Yoga and Physical Exercise - A Review and Comparison." *International Review of Psychiatry* 28 no. 3 (2016): 242-253. doi: 10.3109/09540261.2016.1160878.
4. Tolahunase, M., Sagar, R., Dada, R. "Impact of Yoga and Meditation on Cellular Aging in Apparently Healthy Individuals: A Prospective, Open-Label Single-Arm Exploratory Study." *Oxidative Medicine and Cellular Longevity* 2017 (2017): 9 pages. doi: 10.1155/2017/7928981.
5. Dwivedi, U., et al. "Well-Being at Workplace through Mindfulness: Influence of *Yoga* Practice on Positive Affect and Aggression." *Journal of Research in Ayurveda* 36 no. 4 (2015): 375-379. doi: 10.4103/0974-8520.190693.
6. Deng, G.E., et al. "Evidence-Based Clinical Practice Guidelines for Integrative Oncology: Complementary Therapies and Botanicals." *Journal of the Society for Integrative Oncology* 7 no. 3 (2009): 85-120. PMID: 19706235.
7. Jahnke, R., et al. "A Comprehensive Review of Health Benefits of Qigong and Tai Chi." *American Journal of Health Promotion* 24 no. 6 (2010): e1-e25.
    107. doi: 10.4278/ajhp.081013-LIT-248.
8. Klojcnik, T. "Technology of the Unified Field of Consciousness - Potential Remedy for Solving Problems of the Society." *Informatol* 47 nos. 2-3 (2014) 157-160.
9. Walton, K.G., Schneider, R.H., Nidich, S. "Review of Controlled Research on the Transcendental Meditation Program and Cardiovascular Disease." *Cardiovascular Review* 12 no. 5 (2004): 262-266. doi: 10.1097/01.crd.0000113021.96119.78.

Made in the USA
Middletown, DE
20 February 2018